Great Science Adventures

Discovering the Human Body and Senses

Great Science Adventures is a comprehensive project which is projected to include the titles below. Please check our website, www.greatscienceadventures.com, for updates and product availability.

Great Life Science Studies:
The World of Plants
The World of Insects and Arachnids
Discovering the Human Body and Senses
The World of Vertebrates
Discovering Biomes - Earth's Ecosystems

Great Physical Science Studies:
The World of Tools and Technology
The World of Light and Sound
Discovering Atoms, Molecules, and Matter
Discovering Energy, Forces, and Motion
Discovering Magnets and Electricity

Great Earth Science Studies:
The World of Space
Discovering Earth's Landforms and Surface Features
Discovering Earth's Atmosphere and Weather
Discovering Rocks and Minerals
Discovering Earth's Oceans and Fresh Water

Copyright © 2005 by:
Common Sense Press
8786 Highway 21
Melrose, FL 32666
(352) 475–5757
www.greatscienceadventures.com

Printed in the United States of America
ISBN 1-929683-14-6

The authors and the publisher have made every reasonable effort to ensure that the experiments and activities in this book are safe when performed according to the book's instructions. We assume no responsibility for any damage sustained or caused while performing the activities or experiments in *Great Science Adventures*. We further recommend that students undertake these activities and experiments under the supervision of a teacher, parent, and / or guardian.

Great Science Adventures

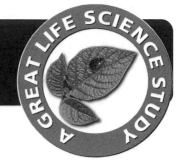

Table of Contents

1. What is the skeletal system? 2

2. What do we know about bones? 4

3. What is the muscular system? 6

4. What do we know about the skin? 10

5. What do we know about hair and nails? 12

6. What do we know about blood? 14

7. What do we know about the heart? 16

8. What is the respiratory system? 20

9. What else do we know about the respiratory system? 22

10. What is the nervous system? 24

11. What do we know about the brain? 28

12. What do we know about sight? 32

13. What do we know about perception? 34

14. What do we know about hearing? 36

15. What do we know about the sense of smell? 40

16. What do we know about the sense of taste? 44

17. What do we know about the sense of touch? 46

18. What is the digestive system? 50

19. What is the urinary system? 54

20. What is the lymphatic system? 56

21. What is the immune system? 58

22. What is the endocrine system? 60

23. What is the reproductive system? 62

24. What do we know about new life? 64

   Lots of Science Library Books 67

   Graphics Pages 143

Great Science Adventures

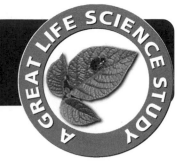

Introduction

Great Science Adventures is a unique, highly effective program that is easy to use for teachers as well as students. This book contains 24 lessons. The concepts to be taught are clearly listed at the top of each lesson. Activities, questions, clear directions, and pictures are included to help facilitate learning. Each lesson will take one to three days to complete.

This program utilizes highly effective methods of learning. Students not only gain knowledge of basic science concepts, but also learn how to apply them.

Specially designed *3D Graphic Organizers* are included for use with the lessons. These organizers review the science concepts while adding to your students' understanding and retention of the subject matter.

This *Great Science Adventures* book is divided into four parts:

1) Following this *Introduction* you will find the *How to Use This Program* section. It contains all the information you need to make the program successful. The *How to Use This Program* section also contains instructions for Dinah Zike's *3D Graphic Organizers*. Please take the time to learn the terms and instructions for these learning manipulatives.

2) In the *Teacher's Section,* the numbered lessons include a list of the science concepts to be taught, simple to complex vocabulary words, and activities that reinforce the science concepts. Each activity includes a list of materials needed, directions, pictures, questions, written assignments, and other helpful information for the teacher.

   The *Teacher's Section* also includes enrichment activities, entitled *Experiences, Investigations, and Research.* Alternative assessment suggestions are found at the end of the *Teacher's Section.*

3) The *Lots of Science Library Books* are next. These books are numbered to correlate with the lessons. Each *Lots of Science Library Book* will cover all the concepts included in its corresponding lesson. You may read the *LSLB* books to your students, ask them to read the books on their own, or make the books available as research materials. Covers for the books are found at the beginning of the *LSLB* section. (Common Sense Press grants permission for you to photocopy the *Lots of Science Library Books* pages and covers for your students.)

4) *Graphic Pages,* also listed by lesson numbers, provide pictures and graphics that can be used with the activities. They can be duplicated and used on student–made manipulatives, or students may draw their own illustrations. The *Investigative Loop* at the front of this section may be photocopied as well. (Common Sense Press grants permission for you to photocopy the *Graphics Pages* for your students.)

Great Science Adventures

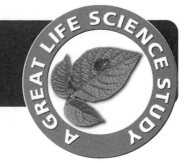

How to Use This Program

This program can be used in a single-level classroom, multilevel classroom, homeschool, co–op group, or science club. Everything you need for a complete tool study is included in this book. Intermediate students will need access to basic reference materials.

Take the time to read the entire *How to Use this Program* section and become familiar with the sections of this book described in the *Introduction*.

Begin a lesson by reading the *Teacher Pages* for that lesson. Choose the vocabulary words for each student and the activities to complete. Collect the materials you need for these activities.

Introduce the lesson with the *Lots of Science Library Book* by reading it aloud or asking a student to read it. (The *Lots of Science Library Books* are located after the *Teacher's Section* in this book.)

Discuss the concepts presented in the *Lots of Science Library Book,* focusing on the ones listed in your *Teacher's Section*.

Follow the directions for the activities you have chosen.

How to Use the Multilevel Approach

The lessons in this book include basic content appropriate for grades K–8 at different mastery levels. For example, throughout the teaching process, a first grader will be exposed to a lot of information but will not be expected to retain all of it. In the same lesson, a sixth-grade student will learn all the steps of the process, be able to communicate them in writing, and be able to apply that information to different situations.

In the *Lots of Science Library Books,* the words written in larger type are for all students. The words in smaller type are for upper level students and include more scientific details about the basic content, as well as interesting facts for older learners.

In the activity sections, icons are used to designate the levels of specific writing assignments.

This icon ✎ indicates the Beginning level, which includes the non-reading or early-reading student. This level applies mainly to kindergarten and first grade students.

This icon ✎✎ is used for the Primary level. It includes the reading student who is still working to be a fluent reader. This level is designed primarily for second and third graders.

This icon ✎✎✎ denotes the Intermediate level, or fluent reader. This level of activities will usually apply to fourth through eighth grade students.

If you are working with a student in seventh or eighth grade, we recommend using the assignments for the Intermediate level, plus at least one *Experiences, Investigations, and Research* activity per lesson.

No matter what grade level your students are working on, use a level of written work that is appropriate for their reading and writing abilities. It is good for students to review data they already know, learn new data and concepts, and be exposed to advanced information and processes.

Vocabulary Words

Each lesson contains a list of vocabulary words used in the content of the lesson. Some of these words will be "too easy" for your students, some will be "too hard," and others will be "just right." The "too easy" words will be used automatically during independent writing assignments. Words that are "too hard" can be used during discussion times. Words that are "just right" can be studied by definition, usage, and spelling. Encourage your students to use these words in their own writing and speaking.

You can encourage beginning students to use their vocabulary words to enhance discussions about the topic and as words to be copied in cooperative writing, or teacher-guided writing.

Primary and Intermediate students can make a Vocabulary Book for new words. Instructions for making a Vocabulary Book are found on page xiii. The Vocabulary Book will contain the word definitions and sentences composed by the student for each word. Students should also be expected to use their vocabulary words in discussions and independent writing assignments. A vocabulary word with an asterisk (*) next to it is designated for Intermediate students only.

Using 3D Graphic Organizers

The *3D Graphic Organizers* provide a format for students of all levels to conceptualize, analyze, review, and apply the concepts of the lesson. The *3D Graphic Organizers* take complicated information and break it down into visual parts so students can better understand the concepts. Most *3D Graphic Organizers* involve writing about the subject matter. Although the content for the levels will generally be the same, assignments and expectations for the levels will vary.

Beginning students may dictate or copy one or two "clue" words about the topic. These students will use the written clues to verbally communicate the science concept. The teacher should provide various ways for the students to restate the concept. This will reinforce the science concept and encourage the students in their reading and higher-order thinking skills.

Primary students may write or copy one or two "clue" words and write a sentence about the topic. The teacher should encourage students to use vocabulary words when writing these sentences. As students read their sentences and discuss the concept, they will reinforce the science concept, increasing their fluency in reading and higher-order thinking skills.

Intermediate students may write several sentences or a paragraph about the topic. These students are also encouraged to use reference materials to expand their knowledge of the subject. As tasks are completed, students enhance their abilities to locate information, read for content, compose sentences and paragraphs, and increase vocabulary. Encourage these students to use the vocabulary words in a context that indicates understanding of the words' meanings.

Illustrations for the *3D Graphic Organizers* are found on the *Graphics Pages* and are labeled by the lesson number and a letter, such as 5–A. Your students may use these graphics to draw their own pictures, or cut out and glue them directly on their work.

Several of the *3D Graphic Organizers* expand over a series of lessons, For this reason, you will need a storage system for each students' *3D Graphic Organizers*. A pocket folder or a reclosable plastic bag works well. See page xi for more information on storing materials.

Investigative Loop™

The *Investigative Loop* is used throughout *Great Science Adventures* to ensure that your labs are effective and practical. Labs give students a context for the application of their science lessons so that they begin to take ownership of the concepts, increasing understanding as well as retention.

The *Investigative Loop* can be used in any lab. The steps are easy to follow, user-friendly, and flexible.

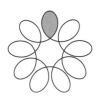 Each *Investigative Loop* begins with a **Question or Concept.** If the lab is designed to answer a question, use a question in this phase. For example, the question could be: "Do muscles need rest to function at their best?" Since the activity for this lab will show that muscles function best after a rest, a question is the best way to begin this *Investigative Loop*.

If the lab is designed to demonstrate a concept, use a concept statement in this phase, such as: "Memory can improve with practice." The lab will demonstrate that fact to the students.

After the **Question or Concept** is formulated, the next phase of the *Investigative Loop* is Research and/or Predictions. Research gives students a foundation for the lab. Having researched the question or concept, students enter the lab with a basis for understanding what they observe. Predictions are best used when the first phase is a question. Predictions can be in the form of a statement, a diagram, or a sequence of events.

The **Procedure** for the lab follows. This is an explanation of how to set up the lab and any tasks involved in it. A list of materials for the lab may be included in this section or may precede the entire *Investigative Loop*.

Whether the lab is designed to answer a question or demonstrate a concept, the students' **Observations** are of prime importance. Instruct the students concerning what they are to focus upon in their observations. The Observation phase will continue until the lab ends.

Once observations are made, students must **Record the Data**. Data may be recorded through diagrams or illustrations. Recording quantitative or qualitative observations about the lab is another important activity in this phase. Records may be kept daily for an extended lab or at the beginning and end for a short lab.

Conclusions and/or Applications are completed when the lab ends. Usually the data records will be reviewed before a conclusion can be drawn about the lab. Encourage the students to defend their conclusions by using the data records. Applications are made by using the conclusions to generalize to other situations or by stating how to use the information in daily life.

Next we must **Communicate the Conclusions**. This phase is an opportunity for students to be creative. Conclusions can be communicated through a graph, story, report, video, mock radio show, etc. Students may also participate in a group presentation.

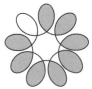

Questions that are asked as the activity proceeds are called **Spark Questions.** Questions that the lab sparks in the minds of the students are important to follow and discuss when the lab ends. The lab itself will answer many of these questions, while others may lead to a new *Investigative Loop*. Assign someone to keep a list of all Spark Questions.

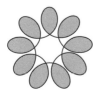

One lab naturally leads to another. This begins a new *Investigative Loop*. The phase called **New Loop** is a brainstorming time for narrowing the lab down to a new question or concept. When the new lab has been decided upon, the *Investigative Loop* begins again with a new Question or Concept.

Take the time to teach your students to make qualitative and quantitative observations. Qualitative observations involve recording the color, texture, shape, smell, size (as small, medium, large), or any words that describe the qualities of an object. Quantitative observations involve using a standard unit of measurement to determine the length, width, weight, mass or volume of an object.

All students will make a Lab Book, in the form of a Large Question and Answer Book, to record information about the Investigative Loops. Instructions are found on page xii. Your students will make a new Lab Book as needed to glue side–by–side to the previous one. Instructions can be found in the *Teacher's Section.* (also xii)

Predictions, data, and conclusions about the *Investigative Loops* are written under the tabs in this book.

When you begin an *Investigative Loop*, ask your students to glue or draw the graphic of the experiment on the tab of the Lab Book. Each *Investigative Loop* is labeled with the lesson number and another number. These numbers are also found on the corresponding graphics.

During an *Investigative Loop*, beginning students should be encouraged to discuss their answers to all experiment questions. By discussing the topic, the students will not only learn the science concepts and procedures, but will be able to organize their thinking in a manner that will assist them in later years of writing. This discussion time is very important for beginning students and should not be rushed.

After the discussion, work with the students to construct a sentence about the topic. Let them copy the sentence. Students can also write "clue" words to help them remember key points about the experiment and discuss it at a later time.

Primary students should be encouraged to verbalize their answers. By discussing the topic, students will learn the science concepts and procedures and learn to organize their thinking, increasing their ability to use higher-level thinking skills. After the discussion, students can complete the assignment using simple phrases or sentences. Encourage students to share the information they have learned with others, such as parents or friends. This will reinforce the content and skills covered in the lesson.

Even though Intermediate students can write the answers to the lab assignments, the discussion process is very important and should not be skipped. By discussing the experiments, students review the science concepts and procedures as well as organize their thinking for the writing assignments. This allows them to think and write at higher levels. These students should be encouraged to use their vocabulary words in their lab writing assignments.

Design Your Own Experiment

After an *Investigative Loop* is completed, intermediate students have the option to design their own experiments based on that lab. The following procedure should be used for those experiments.

Select a Topic based upon an experience in an *Investigative Loop*, science content, an observation, a high-interest topic, a controversial topic, or a current event.

Discuss the Topic as a class, in student groups, and with knowledgeable professionals.

Read and Research the Topic using the library, the Internet, and hands-on investigations and observations, when possible.

Select a Question that can be investigated and answered using easily obtained reference materials, specimens, and/or chemicals, and make sure that the question selected lends itself to scientific inquiry. Ask specific, focused questions instead of broad unanswerable questions. Questions might ask "how" something responds, influences, behaves, determines, forms, or is similar or different to something else.

Predict the answer to your question, and be prepared to accept the fact that your prediction might be incorrect or only partially correct. Examine and record all evidence gathered during testing that both confirms and contradicts your prediction.

Design a Testing Procedure that gathers information that can be used to answer your question. Make sure your procedure results in empirical, or measurable, evidence. Don't forget to do the following:

> Determine where and how the tests will take place – in a natural (field work) or controlled (lab) setting.

> Collect and use tools to gather information and enhance observations.
> Make accurate measurements. Use calculators and computers when appropriate.

> Plan how to document the test procedure and how to communicate and display resulting data.

> Identify variables, or things that might prevent the experiment from being "fair." Before beginning, determine which variables have no effect, a slight effect, or a major effect on your experiment. Create a method for controlling these variables.

Conduct the Experiment carefully and record your findings.

Analyze the Question Again. Determine if the evidence obtained and the scientific explanations of the evidence are reasonable based upon what is known, what you have learned, and what scientists and specialists have reported.

Communicate Findings so that others can duplicate the experiment. Include all pertinent research, measurements, observations, controls, variables, graphs, tables, charts, and diagrams. Discuss observations and results with relevant people.

Reanalyze the Problem and, if needed, redefine the problem and retest. Or, try to apply what was learned to similar problems and situations.

Ongoing Projects: Problem Solving and Inquiry Scenarios

In the Graphic Pages, following the *Investigative Loop,* you will find the Problem Solving and Inquiry Scenarios. Photocopy this page for your students. Allow the students to work on one or more of these scenarios while completing this study of The Human Body and Senses. Although designed for intermediate students, all students may participate if possible.

Experiences, Investigations, and Research

At the end of each lesson in the *Teacher's Section* is a category of activities entitled *Experiences, Investigations, and Research.* These activities expand upon concepts taught in the lesson, provide a foundation for further study of the content, or integrate the study with other disciplines. The following icons are used to identify the type of each activity.

Human Body

Hands On

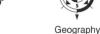

Geography

History

Literature

Math

Research

Writing

Computer

These 3D Graphic Organizers are used throughout Great Science Adventures.

Fast Food and Fast Folds

"If making the manipulatives takes up too much of your instructional time, they are not worth doing. They have to be made quickly, and they can be, if the students know exactly what is expected of them. Hamburgers, Hot Dogs, Tacos, Mountains, Valleys, and Shutter–Folds can be produced by students, who in turn use these folds to make organizers and manipulatives."– Dinah Zike

Every fold has two parts. The outside edge formed by a fold is called the **"Mountain."** The inside of this edge is the **"Valley."**

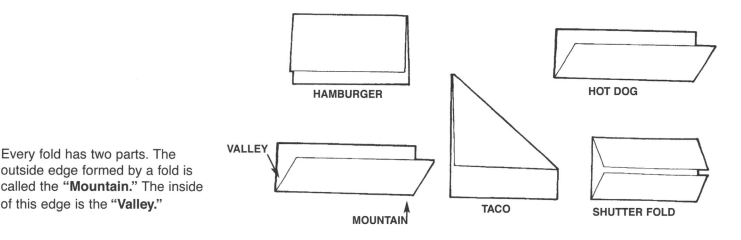

Storage – Book Bags

One–gallon reclosable plastic bags are ideal for storing ongoing projects and books that students are writing and researching.

Use strips of clear, 2" tape to secure 1" x 1" pieces of index card to the front and back of one of the top corners of a bag, under the closure. Punch a hole through the index cards. Use a giant notebook ring to keep several of the "Book Bags" together.

Label the bags by writing on them with a permanent marker.

Alternatively, the bags can be stored in a notebook if you place the 2" clear tape along the side of the storage bag and punch 3 holes in the tape.

Half Book

Fold a sheet of paper in half like a Hamburger.

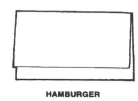

HAMBURGER

Large Question and Answer Book

1. Fold a sheet of paper in half like a Hamburger. Fold it in half again like a Hamburger. Make a cut up the Valley of the inside fold, forming two tabs.

2. A larger book can be made by gluing Large Question and Answer Books "side–by–side."

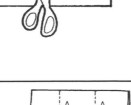

3 Tab Book

1. Fold a sheet of paper in half like a Hamburger or Hot Dog. Fold it into thirds. Cut the inside folds to form three tabs.

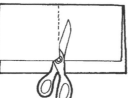

Pocket Book

1. Fold a sheet of paper in half like a Hamburger.

2. Open the folded paper and fold one of the long sides up two and a half–inch inches to form a pocket. Refold along the Hamburger fold so that the newly formed pockets are on the inside.

3. Glue the outer edges of the two and a half–inch fold with a small amount of glue.

4. Make a multi–paged booklet by gluing several Pocket Books "side–by–side."

5. Glue a construction paper cover around the multi–page pocket booklet.

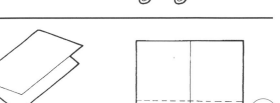

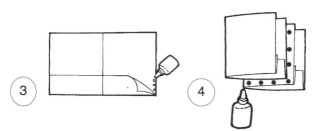

Side–by–Side

Some books can easily grow into larger books by gluing them side–by–side. Make two or more of these books. Be sure the books are closed, then glue the back cover of one book to the front cover of the next book. Continue in this manner, making the book as large as needed. Glue a cover over the whole book.

Layered Look Book

1. Stack two sheets of paper and place the back sheet one inch higher than the front sheet.

2. Bring the bottom of both sheets upward and align the edges so that all of the layers or tabs are the same distance apart.

3. When all tabs are an equal distance apart, fold the papers and crease well.

4. Open the papers and glue them together along the Valley/center fold.

Vocabulary Book

1. Take two sheets of paper and fold each sheet like a Hot Dog.

2. Fold each Hot Dog in half like a Hamburger. Fold each Hamburger in half two more times and crease well. Unfold the sheets of paper, which are divided into sixteenths.

3. On one side only, cut the folds up to the Mountain top, forming eight tabs. Repeat this process on the second sheet of paper.

4. Take a sheet of construction paper and fold like a Hot Dog. Glue the back of one vocabulary sheet to one of the inside sections of the construction paper. Glue the second vocabulary sheet to the other side of the construction paper fold.

5. Vocabulary Books can be made larger by gluing them "side–by–side."

Bound Book

1. Take two sheets of paper and fold each like a Hamburger.

2. Mark both folds 1" from the outer edges.

3. On one of the folded sheets, "cut up" from the top and bottom edge to the marked spot on both sides.

4. On the second folded sheet, start at one of the marked spots and "cut out" the fold between the two marks. Do not cut into the fold too deeply; just shave it off.

5. Take the "cut up" sheet and roll it. Place it through the "cut out" sheet and then open it up. Fold the bound pages in half to form a book.

Variation...
To make a larger book, use additional sheets of paper, marking each sheet as explained in #3. Use an equal number of sheets for the "cut up" and "cut out." Place them one on top of the other and follow the directions in #4 and #5.

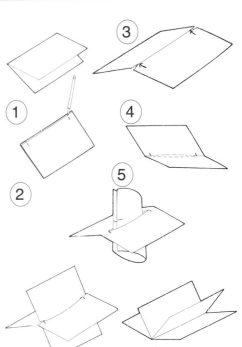

Accordion Book

1. Fold each section of paper into a Hot Dog; however, fold one side 1/2 inch shorter than the other side. This will form a tab that is 1/2 inch long. Fold this tab back away from the shorter piece of paper. Do not fold this tab over the short side, fold it the opposite way.

2. Glue together to form an accordion by gluing a straight edge of one section into the Valley of another section.

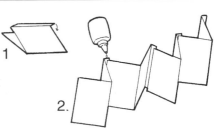

Note: Stand the sections on end and form an accordion with them before gluing. (See illustration.)

5 Top Tab Book _____

1. Make 6 copies of page XV.

2. Cut away squares on each of the pages to make the following:

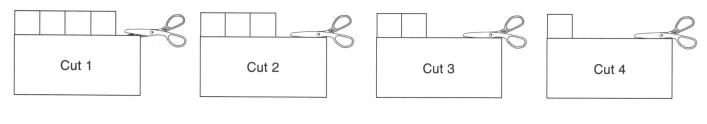

3. Assemble in this order, beginning with the last page.

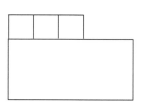

Leave one without cuts to form back page.

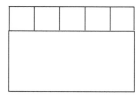

Cut all 5 to form cover.

3. Assemble in this order, beginning with the last page.

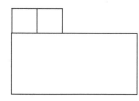

Staple along the left edge.

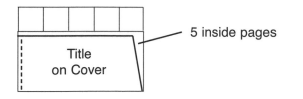

5 inside pages

Title on Cover

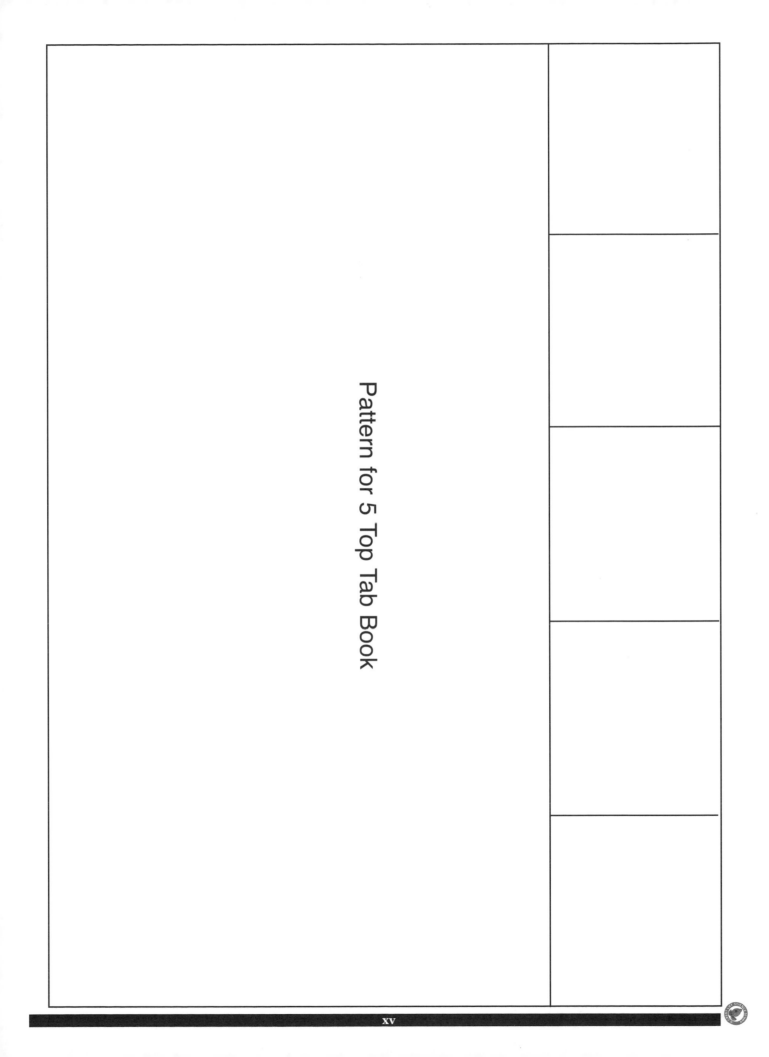

Pattern for 5 Top Tab Book

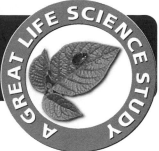

Teacher's Section

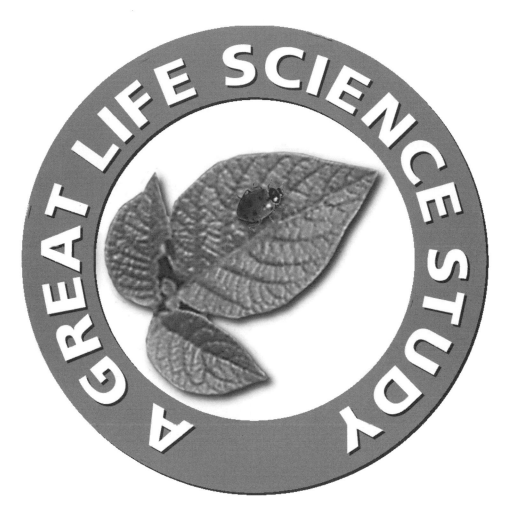

Website addresses used as resources in this book are accurate and relevant at the time of publication. Due to the changing nature of the Internet, we encourage teachers to preview the websites prior to assigning them to students.

The authors and the publisher have made every reasonable effort to ensure that the experiments and activities in this book are safe when performed according to the book's instructions. We further recommend that students undertake these activities and experiments under the supervision of a teacher, parent, or guardian.

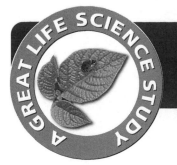

Great Science Adventures

What is the skeletal system?

Human Body Concepts:

- Cells are the building blocks of all living organisms including the human body.
- Groups of similar cells form tissues and tissues form organs.
- Groups of organs working together are called systems.
- The skeletal system is made up of an organized system of bones and cartilage.
- The skeletal system provides support, protects organs, anchors muscles to provide movement, and produces blood cells.
- Two main types of joints are hinge and ball-and-socket.

Vocabulary Words: body   cells   skeleton   joints   *systems   *tissues   *organs
*hinge   *ball-and-socket

Construct and Read: *Lots of Science Library Book #1.* (See page 67)

Activities:

Skeletal System – Graphic Organizer

Focus Skill: explaining a function

Paper Handouts: 12" x 18" sheet of construction paper   8.5" x 11" sheet of paper
   a copy of Graphics 1A - B

Graphic Organizer: Using the 12" x 18" construction paper, make a Shutter Fold. Glue/copy
   Graphic 1A on the left side of the cover as shown. Label the cover of the Shutter Fold
   Skeletal and Muscular Systems. Using the 8.5" x 11" paper, make a Hot Dog. Place
   the Hot Dog so that the fold is on the right side. Glue Graphic 1B on the front and
   label it *Skeletal System*. Open the Shutter Fold and glue the Hot Dog on the left part of
   the middle section, being sure to place the fold on the right side. Open the Hot Dog.
   On the top right side:

✎ Draw a skeleton.

✎✎ Write clue words about the four main functions of the skeletal
   system: *supports the body, protects organs, anchors muscles,
   produces blood cells.*

✎✎✎ Explain the four main functions of the skeletal system.

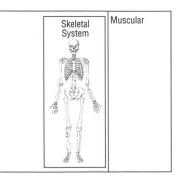

Moveable Joints – Graphic Organizer

Focus Skill: comparing and contrasting

Paper Handouts: 8.5" X 11" sheet of paper   Graphics 1C - F

Graphic Organizer: Make a Hot Dog. Cut it to make a Large Question and Answer Book. Open it so that the Hot Dog's fold is on the left side. Open the *Skeletal and Muscular Systems Shutter Fold.* Glue the Hot Dog on the left section, being sure to place the fold on the left side. Glue/copy Graphics 1C on the top tab and 1D on the bottom tab. Label the tabs *Hinge Joints* and *Ball-and-Socket Joints.* Glue Graphics 1E & 1F under each tab. On the Hinge tab, using a red marker, circle the elbows and knees. On the *Ball-and-Socket* tab, using a blue marker, circle the shoulders and hip joints. Beside the Graphics:

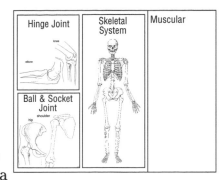

✎ Draw a picture of a hinge joint and a ball-and-socket joint accordingly.

✎✎ Write clue words about each joint and include examples. hinge joint - *move in one direction, strong, elbow and knee.* ball and socket joint - *can be twisted like a joy stick, allows movement in many directions, rotation, shoulder and hip.*

✎✎✎ Describe each joint, explain how they move, and include examples.

This *Skeletal and Muscular Systems Shutter Fold* will be used in Lessons 2-3.

How Tall Are You?

Activity Materials: butcher paper   tape measure

Activity: Lie down on a piece of butcher paper and ask a partner to outline your body. Cut out the outline and fill in the details. Measure the outline.

Experiences, Investigations, and Research

Select one or more of the following activities for individual or group enrichment projects. Allow your students to determine the format in which they would like to report, share, or graphically present what they have discovered. This should be a creative investigation that utilizes your students' strengths.

1. Research the life of Wilhelm Conrad Roentgen and the history of the X-ray, including its uses today.

2. Examine your ears and the tip of your nose. Feel the end of your nose; wiggle it. Bend your ear. Can you do this with parts of your body such as your finger tips or toes? Why or why not?

3. Use modeling clay to make a stand-up figure. Make another figure using toothpicks as a frame. Cover the frame with clay. Which figure holds its shape better?

4. Read *Clara Barton, Founder of the American Red Cross* (The Childhood of Famous Americans Series) by Augusta Stevenson. ✎✎ & ✎✎✎

5. http://www.bartleby.com/107/ - Use this site throughout the study to view colored illustrations on the human body. ✎✎✎

6. http://bart.northnet.com.au/~amcgann/body/

7. http://library.thinkquest.org/10348/- Contains various systems; ideal for ✎✎ & ✎✎✎

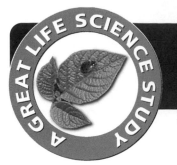

What do we know about bone?

Human Body Concepts:

- Bone tissue is made up of living cells.
- Bones are lightweight yet strong.
- Bone's three layers consist of a tough outer layer, compact bone, and spongy bone.
- Red bone marrow produces all red blood cells and some white blood cells.
- A fracture may be simple, complete, compound, or other.

Vocabulary Words: bones   calcium   *cartilage   *compact bone   *spongy bone
*red bone marrow   *fracture

Construct and Read: *Lots of Science Library Book #2.*

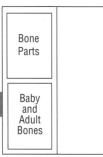

Activities:

Bone Parts – Graphic Organizer

Focus Skill: comparing and contrasting
Paper Handouts: 8.5" x 11" sheet of paper   a copy of Graphic 2A
    Skeletal and Muscular Systems Shutter Fold

Graphic Organizer: Make a Hot Dog. Place the Hot Dog in front of you so that the fold is on top. Glue/copy Graphic 2A on the front of the Hot Dog. Cut the Hot Dog to make a 3 Tab Book. Fold over the right and left tabs and label the cover *Bone Parts*. Open the *Skeletal and Muscular Systems Shutter Fold*. Open the *Skeletal System* book. Keeping the 3 Tab Book folded, glue it on the top left side. Open the 3 Tab Book so you are looking at Graphic 2A. Label the left tab *Outer Layer*. Label the middle tab *Compact Bone*. Label the *Spongy Bone* tab.

- ✎ Color the spongy bone in brown, color the compact bone white, and the outer layer in light brown.
- ✎✎ Open the tabs. Write clue words about each part of the bone. outer layer - *tough membrane, nerves, blood vessels, special cells help repair bone injuries.* compact bones - *bone cells release minerals, very strong, have holes and channels to carry blood vessels and nerves to inner bone.* spongy bone - *at end of bone, spongy looking, tiny pieces of bones, looks like honeycomb, hollow spaces filled with bone marrow.*
- ✎✎✎ Open the tabs. Describe each part of the bone and define its function.

Baby and Adult Bones – Graphic Organizer

Focus Skill: comparing and contrasting
Paper Handouts: 8.5" x 11" sheet of paper   a copy of Graphics 2B-C
Graphic Organizer: Make a Large Question and Answer Book. Label the cover *Baby Bones* and *Adult Bones*. Glue this in the *Skeletal and Muscular Systems Shutter Fold*, in the *Skeletal System* book, beneath the Bone *Parts* Graphic Organizer. Open the tabs.

✎ Under the *Baby* tab, draw a picture of yourself when you were a baby. Under the *Adult* tab, draw a picture of an adult. Circle the nose and ears to help you remember the parts that remain as cartilage.

✎✎ Under the *Baby* tab, write clue words about a baby's bones. Under the *Adult* tab, write clue words about an adult's bones. baby bones - *minerals make bones harder, bone tissues develop at center and grow.* adult bones - *can become brittle and break easily.*

✎✎✎ Under each tab, compare and contrast a baby's bones to an adult's bones. Define cartilage and list areas of the body that remain as cartilage throughout an adult's life. (Refer to *Lots of Science Library Book #1* and *2*.)

Bending Bones

Activity Materials: chicken leg bone   vinegar   bowl
Activity: Take a chicken leg bone and put it in a bowl filled with vinegar. Leave it for two to three days. Pour away the vinegar, wash the bone with water and then try to bend it. How does it feel? Why? **The bone bends because the acidic vinegar has dissolved the calcium in it.**

All Thumbs

Activity Materials: tape
Activity: Tape your partner's thumbs down on the palm, leaving the remaining fingers free. Record your observations as your partner tries to eat, write, use the telephone, and do other activities. Trade places with your partner. Explain the importance of the skeletal structure in the hand, fingers, and thumbs in everyday activities.

Experiences, Investigations, and Research

Select one or more of the following activities for individual or group enrichment projects. Allow your students to determine the format in which they would like to report, share, or graphically present what they have discovered. This should be a creative investigation that utilizes your students' strengths.

1. Research food labels. Discover which foods are high in calcium and explain why this is important.

2. Research osteoporosis. Answer the questions: What are the causes? Who is afflicted the most? Is there a way to prevent it? Is treatment available?

3. Read *A Picture Book of Florence Nightingale* by David A. Adler. ✎ ✎✎

4. Read *Florence Nightingale* (Young Reader's Christian Library Series) by Kristi Lorene. ✎✎✎

5. http://www.howstuffworks.com/cell.htm

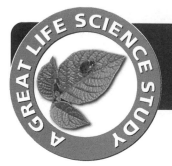

What is the
muscular system?

Human Body Concepts:

- Muscles are necessary for body movements.
- The three types of muscles are skeletal, smooth, and cardiac.
- Skeletal muscles are attached to bones and work in pairs.
- Smooth muscles are located in the walls of organs, arteries, and eyes.
- Cardiac muscles are found in the heart.
- The more a muscle works, the more oxygen it needs.

Vocabulary Words: muscles   pairs   contracts   oxygen   *ligaments

*involuntary   *voluntary

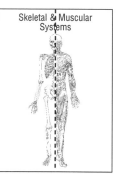

Construct and Read: *Lots of Science Library Book #3.*

Activities:

Muscular System – Graphic Organizer

Focus Skill: defining terms
Paper Handouts: 8.5" x 11" sheet of paper   a copy of Graphics 3A - B
   Skeletal and Muscular Systems Shutter Fold
Graphic Organizer: Glue 3A on the right side of the cover of the *Skeletal and Muscular Systems Shutter Fold.* Make a Hot Dog. Glue/copy Graphic 3B on the cover and label it *Muscular System.* Open the *Skeletal and Muscular Systems Shutter Fold.* Glue the Hot Dog in the middle section beside the *Skeletal System*, being sure to keep the fold on the left side. Open the Hot Dog.

✎   Draw a picture that shows you using your muscles.

✎✎   Write clue words about the muscular system. *human skeleton is covered with over 600 muscles, muscles make bones move, muscles need good food and exercise.*

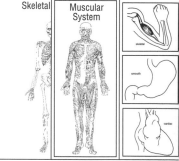

✎✎✎   Define muscles, ligaments, and tendons. Compare and contrast voluntary and involuntary muscles and give examples of each.

Three Types of Muscles – Graphic Organizer

Focus Skill: *describing*
Paper Handouts: 8.5" x 11" sheet of paper   a copy of Graphics 3C - E
Graphic Organizer: Make a Hot Dog 3 Tab Book with the fold on the
   right side. Glue/copy Graphics 3C - E on each tab. Label it *Three Types of Muscles.*
   Label each tab *Cardiac Muscle, Skeletal Muscle,* and *Smooth Muscle* accordingly. Open
   the *Skeletal and Muscular Systems Shutter Fold.* Glue the *Three Types of Muscles Graphic
   Organizer* on the right side. Open the tabs.

✎ On the *Cardiac* tab, draw a heart; on the *Skeletal* tab, draw muscle attached to a bone; on the *Smooth* tab, draw a blood vessel.

✎✎ Under each tab, write clue words about each type of muscle. skeletal muscles - *you control these muscles, used to move, are long, thin, strands.* smooth muscles - *found in walls of internal organs and arteries, you do not control.* cardiac muscles - *in the heart, strong, works 24 hours a day.*

✎✎✎ Under each tab, describe each muscle and list examples.

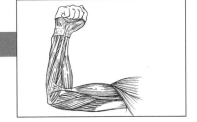

Investigative Loop - Muscles Need Rest

Focus Skill: predicting an outcome

Lab Materials: watch with a second hand

Paper Handouts: 8.5" x 11" sheet of paper
  Lab Record Cards (index cards or 1/4 sheets of paper)
  Lab Graphic 3-1

Graphic Organizer: Make a Pocket Book. This is the student's Lab Book. In future lessons, Pocket Books will be made and glued side-by-side to this one. Glue Lab Graphic 3-1 on the left pocket.

Question: Do muscles need rest to function at their best?

Research: Read *Lots of Science Library Book #3* and review what you know about muscles.

Prediction: Predict whether muscles perform better after rest. Write your prediction on a Lab Record Card labeled "Lab 3-1."

Procedure: Make a fist and open it with fingers extended. Do this as many times as you can within 15 seconds. With no rest in between, complete this 5 more times. Take a 15-minute rest period. Clench and unclench your fist 5 more times.

Observations: Make quantitative observations to compare muscles before and after rest.

Record the Data: Label a Lab Record Card "Lab 3-1." Record the data after the first session of opening and closing your fist. Record the data after each of the 5 sessions. Record the data after the 15-minute rest.

Conclusions: Explain why your performance differed from the first session through to the last session. Draw conclusions about the relationship between muscles and rest.

Communicate the Conclusions: Write your conclusions on a Lab Record Card labeled "Lab 3-1." Compare your observations and conclusions with your predictions. Share your Lab Record Cards with one person who did not participate in the Lab. Place the Lab Record Cards in the Lab Book for Lab 3-1.

Spark Questions: Discuss questions sparked by this lab.

New Loop: Choose one question to investigate further. Or, repeat the same procedure using a different activity or a shorter or longer rest period.

Muscle Power

Activity: Sit in front of a table. Place one hand under the table, palm up. Press up on the table. With your free hand, feel the biceps and triceps in your working arm. Now, place your hand on top of the table, palm up. Press down on the table and feel your biceps and triceps. When you pressed up on the table, which muscle was harder, the biceps or triceps? **The biceps was harder.** When you pressed down on the table, which muscle was harder? **The triceps was harder.**

Voluntary and Involuntary Muscles

Activity: Raise your right arm. Extend your left arm. Jump. In these activities, do your muscles move on their own (involuntary), or did you decide to make them move (voluntary)? Now, place your hand over your heart. Can you feel your heart beating? Is your cardiac muscle moving on its own or do you decide to make it move? Discuss similarities and differences between arm muscles and cardiac muscles.

Tendons

Activity Materials: chicken leg with foot (available from a butcher)   tweezers
Activity: Locate the tendons at the top of the leg. They look like cords. Using tweezers, pull one tendon. What happened? **The foot will move**.

Experiences, Investigations, and Research

Select one or more of the following activities for individual or group enrichment projects. Allow your students to determine the format in which they would like to report, share, or graphically present what they have discovered. This should be a creative investigation that utilizes your students' strengths.

1. Make a list of voluntary and involuntary muscles.

2. Read *The Magic School Bus: Inside the Human Body* by Joanna Cole.

3. http://www.howstuffworks.com/sports-physiology10.htm

Notes

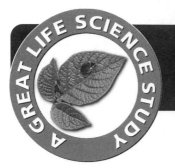

What do we know about the skin?

Human Body Concepts:

- The skin, hair, and nails are the integumentary system.
- Skin's three layers are epidermis, dermis, and subcutaneous tissue.
- The epidermis is the outer layer of skin that is made up of dead cells.
- The dermis, located beneath the epidermis, is strong and stretchy.
- The dermis contains sensory nerves, blood vessels, sweat glands, and oil glands.
- Skin senses touch, pain, and temperature.
- Skin helps maintain body temperature.

Vocabulary Words: skin dermis epidermis *integumentary *keratin
*melanin *subcutaneous

Construct and Read: *Lots of Science Library Book #4.*

Integumentary System
Nails
Hair
Skin

Activities:

Parts of the Skin – Graphic Organizer

Focus Skill: labeling

Paper Handouts: 2 sheets of 8.5" x 11" paper   a copy of Graphics 4A - B

Graphic Organizer: Make a Layered Look Book. Label the cover *Integumentary System.* From the bottom tab to the top tab, label them *Skin, Hair, Nails.* Open it to the *S*kin tab. Glue/copy Graphic 4A on bottom section. Label the parts of the skin: *epidermis, dermis, subcutaneous tissue.*

✎ Color the epidermis pink, dermis orange, and subcutaneous tissue yellow.

✎✎ On the top right section, write clue words about skin: *protects the body, feels touch, pain, temperature, keeps body at 98.6°, protects from germs.*

✎✎✎ On the top section, define the three parts of skin and explain its four main functions.

Melanin

Turn to the *Skin* tab of the *Integumentary System Layered Look Book.* Glue/copy Graphic 4B on the top left section. Label it *Melanin.* Below each Graphic:

✎ Draw a picture of a boy/girl with little melanin and a picture of a boy/girl with larger amounts of melanin.

✎✎ Write clue words about melanin in the skin: *pigment that decides skin color and absorbs sunlight, little melanin = fair skinned, large amounts melanin = darker skin.*

✎✎✎ Define melanin and its purpose.

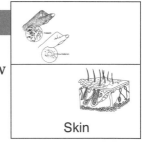

Skin

This *Integumentary System Layered Look Book* will be used in Lesson 5.

Cool Sweat

Activity Materials: 2 cotton balls   rubbing alcohol   water

Activity: Soak one cotton ball with water and the other cotton ball with rubbing alcohol. Rub the water cotton ball on the inside of one wrist; rub the alcohol cotton ball on the other wrist. What happens to the water and alcohol on your wrists? **They evaporate.** Which is evaporating quicker? **Alcohol** Which wrist feels cooler? **Alcohol** How does perspiration cool the body? **As sweat evaporates, it releases heat energy.**

A Close Look at Skin

Activity Materials: magnifying glass

Activity: Look at your skin through a magnifying glass. What part of the skin are you looking at? **Epidermis** What kind of cells make up this layer? **Dead cells** Locate the tiny hairs and their openings. Locate the tiny sweat pores. Gently rub or scratch the skin on your arm. Do you see dead skin cells?

Sweat Glands

Activity Materials: iodine   water   cornstarch   sheet of white paper cotton ball

Activity: Cut the sheet of paper into 2-inch squares. Mix 2 teaspoons of cornstarch into 1/2 cup of water. Stir. Dip the paper squares into the cornstarch solution and set aside to dry. Using a cotton ball, apply iodine to the palm of your hand. Run up and down stairs or run on the spot to begin perspiring. Place the cornstarch paper on your palm and press down. What do you see? **Sweat glands should appear as dark spots.**

Experiences, Investigations, and Research

Select one or more of the following activities for individual or group enrichment projects. Allow your students to determine the format in which they would like to report, share, or graphically present what they have discovered. This should be a creative investigation that utilizes your students' strengths.

1. Find a partner(s). Press your finger on an ink pad and with a gentle, rolling motion make a fingerprint on paper. Examine your fingerprint and your partner's fingerprint. Observe the patterns and compare and contrast the two prints. Investigate why fingerprints are helpful in police work.

2. Learn to take your temperature. Wipe the thermometer with rubbing alcohol and rinse with cold water. Shake the thermometer to bring the reading to less than 96 degrees. Place the bulb under your tongue for 3 minutes. Sit and do not talk. What is your normal temperature? Take your temperature at different times of the day: after a hot shower, after a cold shower, after a run, or in the morning. Draw conclusions from this investigation.

3. http://www.howstuffworks.com/sunscreen.htm

4. http://www.howstuffworks.com/sweat.htm

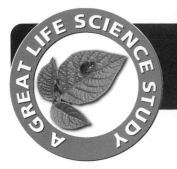

What do we know about hair and nails?

Human Body Concepts:

- Hair is made of a string of overlapping dead cells along with keratin that adds to hair's strength.
- A hair follicle contains melanin which gives hair its color.
- A round follicle grows straight hair; an oval follicle grows wavy hair; a flat follicle grows curly hair.
- Nails are made up of dead cells.
- Nails are strong because they consist of keratin.

Vocabulary Words: hair nails curly wavy straight round oval flat
*hair follicle   *nail plate

Construct and Read: *Lots of Science Library Book #5.*

Activities:

Straight, Wavy, and Curly Hair – Graphic Organizer

Focus Skill: comparing and contrasting
Paper Handouts: a copy of Graphics 5A - C   *Integumentary System Layered Look Book*
Graphic Organizer: Turn to the *Hair* tab in the *Integumentary System Layered Look Book*.
Glue/copy Graphic 5A on the top of the bottom section. On each Graphic, draw the type of follicle each type of hair grows from. Below the Graphics:

✎ Draw a person with straight hair, wavy hair, and curly hair, accordingly.

✎✎ Write clue words about each type of hair and hair follicle: round – *straight hair;* oval – *wavy hair;* flat – *curly.* Label the pictures *Straight, Wavy,* and *Curly.*

✎✎✎ Explain the relationship of the shape of the hair follicle to the type of hair.

Hair Up Close

Turn to the *Hair* tab of the *Integumentary System Layered Look Book*. Glue/copy Graphic 5B on the top left section. Label it *Hair Up Close*. On the left side:

✎ Look in the mirror and draw yourself paying close attention to your hair.

✎✎ Write clue words about the structure of hair and its purpose. *body covered with hair, hair on head keeps head warm and protects from the sun, eyebrows and eyelashes keep dirt from eyes, hair is a string of dead cells that overlap, keratin adds strength to hair, a living root pushes the strand.*

✎✎✎ Explain the structure of hair and list the factors that make hair strong. Define the purpose of hair.

Nails

Turn to the *Nail* tab of the *Integumentary System Layered Look Book*. Glue/copy Graphic 5C on the bottom section. Label the parts of the nail: *nail plate* and *nail root*. On the top section:

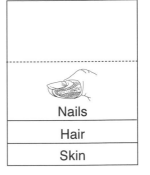

Nails

Hair

Skin

✏️ Trace your hand or fingers. Draw nails on the fingers.

✏️✏️ Write clue words about nails: *nails are made of keratin, visible part is the nail plate made of dead cells and grows from a nail root.*

✏️✏️✏️ Describe nails. Include information on growth rate and composition.

This completes your Integumentary System Layered Look Book. Present it to at least one person and tell them everything you have learned about human skin, hair, and nails.

Hair Up Close

Activity Materials: magnifying glass

Activity: Hold a strand of hair close to the root and with a firm, quick motion, pull a hair with its root intact. Look at the hair shaft with a magnifying glass; look at the root. Describe what you see. Hold one end of the strand of hair. Run your thumb and index finger down to the tip. How does it feel? Hold it upside down and repeat. How does it feel? Was there a difference? Why?

Experiences, Investigations, and Research

Select one or more of the following activities for individual or group enrichment projects. Allow your students to determine the format in which they would like to report, share, or graphically present what they have discovered. This should be a creative investigation that utilizes your students' strengths.

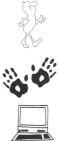

1. Put a dot of nail polish on one fingernail and one toenail. Leave it for several weeks. Check it during that time and reapply as it fades. Compare the growth of your fingernail and toenail.

2. Try picking up a dime without using your fingernails. Can you do it?

3. http://www.howstuffworks.com/hair-coloring1.htm

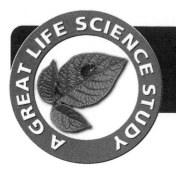

What do we know about blood?

Human Body Concepts:

- Blood is the only liquid tissue. It is part of the cardiovascular system.
- Blood transports nutrients and wastes, regulates body temperature, and protects the body after an injury and against disease.
- Blood consists of red blood cells, white blood cells, and platelets.
- Red blood cells carry oxygen to all body cells.
- White blood cells protects the body from germs and other harmful agents.
- Platelets help blood to clot.

Vocabulary Words: blood   clot   carbon dioxide   *cardiovascular   *plasma
*platelets   *hemoglobin

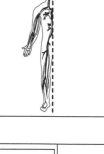

Cardiovascular and Respiratory Systems

Construct and Read: *Lots of Science Library Book #6.*

Activities:

Cardiovascular System – Graphic Organizer

Focus Skills: explaining functions
Paper Handouts: 12" x 18" construction paper   8.5" x 11" sheet of paper
    a copy of Graphics 6A - B

Graphic Organizer: Using the 12" x 18" construction paper, make a Shutter Fold. Glue/copy Graphic 6A on the cover as shown. Label the Shutter Fold *Cardiovascular and Respiratory Systems*. Using the 8.5" x 11" sheet of paper, make a Hot Dog. Lay the Hot Dog so the fold is on the right side.

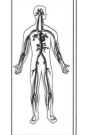

Glue/copy Graphic 6B on the front and label it *Cardiovascular System*. Open the *Cardiovascular and Respiratory Systems Shutter Fold* and glue the *Cardiovascular System* on the left side of the middle section. Open the *Cardiovascular System*. On the top right side:

✎ Draw an outline of your body. Using a red marker, draw blood vessels and the heart.

✎✎ Write clue words about the three main functions of blood. *1. carries oxygen from lungs to the body, carries carbon dioxide from body to lungs to be exhaled, carries nutrients from stomach and intestines to body, and carries wastes out of body. 2. keeps body temperature at 98.6°. 3. Helps stop bleeding, protects body from disease.*

✎✎✎ Explain the three main functions of blood. Research the different blood types and the need for blood donors.

Focus Skill: explaining a process
Paper Handouts: 8.5" x 11" sheet of paper   a copy of Graphic 6C - F
Graphic Organizer: Make a Hot Dog and cut along the valley. (Save one strip for Lesson 18.)
    Make an Accordion Book. Place the Accordion Book so that the folds are on the left
    side. Label it *Clot*. Open the Accordion Book and glue/copy Graphics 6C - F on the top
    of each section. Open the *Cardiovascular and Respiratory Systems Shutter Fold*, open
    the *Cardiovascular System*. Close the Accordion and glue it on the bottom right section.
    On each tab of the Accordion:
✎   Write 1, 2, 3, 4.
✎✎ ✎✎✎ Write about the clotting process. *1. A cut*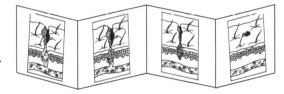
occurs in the skin. 2. Platelets quickly collect at the cut
to prevent excessive loss of blood. 3. A clot of thick
blood forms. White blood cells destroy harmful bacteria.
4. The clot dries, a scab is formed, allowing time for the
tissue to repair itself.

Experiences, Investigations, and Research

Select one or more of the following activities for individual or group enrichment projects.
Allow your students to determine the format in which they would like to report, share, or
graphically present what they have discovered. This should be a creative investigation that
utilizes your students' strengths.

1. http://www.howstuffworks.com/heart3.htm

2. http://www.howstuffworks.com/heart5.htm

3. Investigate the following and record the results of your investigation:
    a. How many quarts of blood are in the human body?
    b. What is a "blood bank"?
    c. When and why do people need blood transfusions?
    d. What diseases can be carried by blood?
    e. How are blood supplies kept safe?

4. What type of blood do your parents have? Explain blood types and
    their importance.

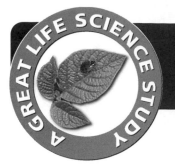

What do we know about the heart?

Human Body Concepts:

- The cardiovascular system consists of blood, the heart, and blood vessels.
- Arteries carry oxygen-rich blood from the heart to all body cells.
- Veins carry deoxygenated blood back to the heart.
- The heart is a hollow organ made up of two pumps working together.
- The harder the body works, the faster the heart pumps to receive more oxygen and release carbon dioxide.

Vocabulary Words: heart   pump   arteries   veins   pulse   circulate
*blood vessels   *capillaries   *aorta   *valves   *atrium   *ventricle

Construct and Read: *Lots of Science Library Book #7.*

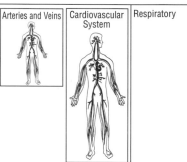

Activities:

Blood Vessels – Graphic Organizer

Focus Skills: *explaining functions*
Paper Handouts: 8.5" x 11" sheet of paper   a copy of Graphics 7A
    Cardiovascular and Respiratory Systems Shutter Fold
Graphic Organizer: Make a Hot Dog with the fold on the left side. Cut it into a 2 Tab Book. Glue/copy Graphics 7A on the top tab. Label it *Arteries* and *Veins*. Open the *Cardiovascular and Respiratory Systems Shutter Fold* and glue the Hot Dog on the left side. Use red highlighter to trace the arteries to show oxygen-rich blood. Use a blue highlighter to trace the veins to show deoxygenated blood. Open the tab:

✎ Draw a picture of your body with veins and arteries.

✎✎ Write clue words about veins and arteries. veins – *take oxygen-depleted blood to heart, thin wall, valves to prevent blood from flowing backward.* arteries – *strong, thick walls, muscular, elastic, take oxygen-filled blood to body.*

✎✎✎ Describe veins and arteries and define their functions.

The Human Heart - Graphic Organizer

Focus Skills: labeling
Paper Handouts: 8.5" x 11" sheet of paper   a copy of Graphics 7B - C
    Cardiovascular and Respiratory Systems Shutter Fold
Graphic Organizer: Glue Graphic 7B on the bottom tab, under the Veins and Arteries tab. Label it *Heart*. Glue/copy Graphic 7C inside. Open the *Heart* tab.

- ✎ Color the atrium orange; ventricle pink; aorta red
- ✎✎ Label the parts of the heart: *right atrium, left atrium, right ventricle, left ventricle, pulmonary artery, aorta.*
- ✎✎✎ Complete ✎✎. Explain how blood moves throughout the body.

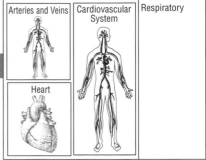

Investigative Loop – Pulsating Heart

Focus Skill: *predicting an outcome*
Lab Materials: stairs or low stool   watch with a minute hand
Paper Handouts: Lab Book   Lab Record Cards
    Lab Graphic 7-1
Graphic Organizer: Glue Lab Graphic 7-1 on the right pocket of the Lab Book.
Question: Does physical activity affect heart rate?
Research: Read *Lots of Science Library Book #7* and review what you know about the heart and blood vessels.

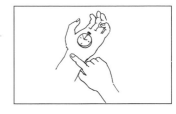

Prediction: Predict whether physical activity will affect your heart rate. Record your prediction on a Lab Record Card labeled "Lab 7-1."
Procedure: In a resting state, take your pulse. Now, step up and down on a stair or stool quickly 10 times. Allow a few minutes for rest and complete the activity again, stepping up and down 20 times. Take your pulse. Rest. Now step 30 times. Take your pulse.
Observations: Observe your pulse during the resting state and after each session of activity.
Record the Data: On a Lab Record Card labeled "Lab 7-1," record your pulse rate during the resting state and after each session of stair stepping. Recording the data must be done immediately; or have a partner record the data.
Conclusions: Draw conclusions about how activity affects heart rate. To complete this activity, your leg muscles require more oxygen. Oxygen is carried in the blood, so the heart beats faster to pump more blood to the muscles.
Communicate the Conclusions: On another Lab Record Card labeled "Lab 7-1," write your conclusions. Compare your observations and conclusions with your predictions. Share your Lab Record Cards with one person who did not participate in the Lab. Place the Lab Record Cards in the Lab Book for Lab 7-1.
Spark Questions: Discuss questions sparked by this lab.
New Loop: Choose one question to investigate further. Or, complete the same procedure with a variety of participants (various ages, weights, male/female). Compare and contrast.

Mighty Pumping Heart

Activity Materials: tennis ball
Activity: Squeeze a tennis ball in your hand 70 times a minute. This shows about how hard your heart works.

Viewing Blood Vessels

Activity: Two good places to observe living blood vessels are under your tongue and in the fold under your eye. Look in the mirror and curl up your tongue. Can you see the blood vessels? What color are they? What kind of blood vessels are the blue lines? **Veins.** What kind of blood vessels are the pink lines? **Arteries.**

Experiences, Investigations, and Research

Select one or more of the following activities for individual or group enrichment projects. Allow your students to determine the format in which they would like to report, share, or graphically present what they have discovered. This should be a creative investigation that utilizes your students' strengths.

1. Visit your local butcher and request a lamb heart. (A lamb's heart is similar to a human heart in shape and size.) Try to identify the main blood vessels. Slice the heart in half and locate the chambers, valves, arteries, and veins.

2. Research the relationship between the heart and aerobic exercise, and the relationship between the heart and good nutrition.

3. Locate a stethoscope. Listen to your heartbeat; listen to your partner's heartbeat. If possible, listen to the heartbeat of people of various ages and compare your findings.

4. Many pharmacies have blood pressure machines for public use. Check your blood pressure. Compare it with others.

5. Research the medical contributions of Christiaan Barnard and the first human heart transplant. Compare early heart transplants to those performed today.

6. http://www.howstuffworks.com/heart.htm

7. http://www.merck.com/disease/heart/coronary_health/anatomy/home.html

Notes

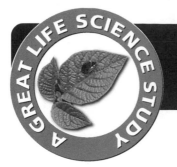
What is the respiratory system?

Human Body Concepts:

- The body needs oxygen to break down food and release stored energy.
- The respiratory system consists of the mouth, nose, trachea, and lungs.
- Lungs are the main organs within the respiratory system.
- The trachea divides into two airways that lead to the lungs.
- Each lung contains airways, air sacs, and blood vessels.

Vocabulary Words: air   breathe   lungs   *respiratory   *trachea   *lobes

*air sacs   *bronchi

Construct and Read: *Lots of Science Library Book #8.*

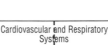

Activities:

Look at Lungs - Graphic Organizer

Focus Skills: labeling
Paper Handouts: 8.5" x 11" sheet of paper   a copy of Graphic 8A - C
Cardiovascular and Respiratory Systems Shutter Fold
Graphic Organizer: Glue Graphic 8A on the right side of *Cardiovasular and Respiratory Systems Shutter Fold.* Make a Hot Dog with the fold on the left side. Glue/copy Graphic 8B on the front. Label it *Respiratory System.* Glue it on the right side of the middle section inside the *Cardiovascular and Respiratory Systems Shutter Fold.* Glue/copy Graphic 8C inside the Hot Dog. Draw your head at the top connected to the trachea.

✎ With a blue highlighter, trace the respiratory system.

✎✎ Label the parts of the respiratory system: *nose, mouth, trachea, right lung, left lung.*

✎✎✎ Label the parts of the respiratory system: *nose; mouth; trachea; bronchi; bronchioles; right lung and its superior, middle, and inferior lobes; left lung and its superior and inferior lobes. Explain the respiratory process.*

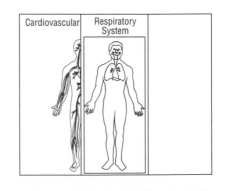

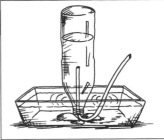

Focus Skill: following directions

Lab Materials: 2 liter bottle   2 feet of rubber tubing (from craft store)   large pan of water   permanent marker

Paper Handouts: 8.5" x 11" sheet of paper   Record Cards   Lab Book   Lab Graphic 8-1

Graphic Organizer: Make a Pocket Book and glue it side-by-side to the existing Lab Book. Glue Lab Graphic 8-1 on the left pocket of the new Pocket Book.

Question: Is there a difference in lung capacity during normal breathing and deep breathing?

Research: Read *Lots of Science Library Book #8* and review what you know about lungs.

Prediction: Predict whether there is a difference between normal breathing and deep breathing. Record your prediction on a Lab Record Card labeled "8-1."

Procedure: Fill a large pan half full of water. Fill a bottle with water almost to the top. Place your hand over the top of the jug and invert it into the pan of water. Ask someone to hold the bottle in place. Place one end of the rubber tubing in the bottle. Mark the top of the waterline with a marker. Breathing normally, inhale and hold. Place the tube in your mouth and exhale normally. Mark the top of the waterline. Set up the activity again using the same amount of water. Now, take in a deep breath, hold it, and place the tube in your mouth. Exhale until you cannot exhale any longer. Mark the top of the waterline.

Observations: Make quantitative observations by looking at the line when you exhaled normally. Look at the line when you exhaled deeply.

Record the Data: On another Lab Record Card labeled "Lab 8-1," record your observations. Sketch a picture of the jar and its markings after each exhalation.

Conclusions: Draw conclusions about normal breathing, deep breathing, and lung capacity.

Communicate the Conclusions: On another Lab Record Card labeled "Lab 8-1," compare your observations and conclusions with your predictions. Share your Lab Record Cards with one person who did not participate in the Lab. Store them in the Lab Book for Lab 8-1.

Spark Questions: Discuss questions sparked by this lab.

New Loop: Choose one question to investigate further. Or, complete the same procedure with participants of various ages. Compare the data.

Experiences, Investigations, and Research

Select one or more of the following activities for individual or group enrichment projects. Allow your students to determine the format in which they would like to report, share, or graphically present what they have discovered. This should be a creative investigation that utilizes your students' strengths.

1. Interview someone who does aerobic exercises, such as jogging or swimming. Discover why exercise programs started, why they continue, and what benefits are received from aerobic exercise. Describe and compare different types of exercise programs.

2. Begin your own physical fitness program with advice from a knowledgeable adult.

3. http://www.howstuffworks.com/lung.htm

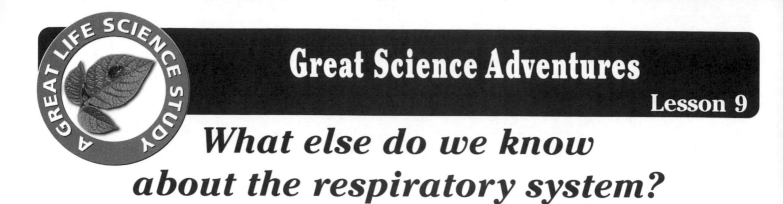

What else do we know about the respiratory system?

Human Body Concepts:

- When you inhale, air enters the nose, moves down the trachea, splits into two airways, and enters the right and left lungs.
- When you exhale, you release carbon dioxide.
- The cardiovascular and respiratory systems work together to carry oxygen to all body cells and remove carbon dioxide.

Vocabulary Words: inhale exhale waste remove energy rest *gas exchange *diaphragm

Construct and Read: *Lots of Science Library Book #9.*

Activities:

Respiratory System – Graphic Organizer

Focus Skills: explaining a process
Paper Handouts: 8.5" x 11" sheet of paper   *Lungs* Graphic Organizer from Lesson 8
   Cardiovascular and Respiratory Systems Shutter Fold
Graphic Organizer: Open the *Cardiovascular and Respiratory Systems Shutter Fold.* On the under side of the *Respiratory System* book:

✎ Draw a picture of yourself resting and a picture of yourself running.
✎✎ Complete ✎.
✎✎✎ Explain the respiratory system using your vocabulary words.

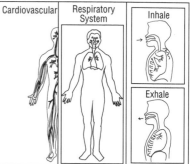

Inhale and Exhale - Graphic Organizer

Focus Skills: *comparing and contrasting*
Paper Handouts: 8.5" x 11" sheet of paper   a copy of Graphics 9A - B
Graphic Organizer: Make a Hot Dog Large Question and Answer Book. Lay the Hot Dog with the fold on the right side. Glue/copy Graphics 9A - B on each tab. Label the tabs *Inhale* and *Exhale* accordingly. Open the *Cardiovascular and Respiratory Systems Shutter Fold.* Glue the *Inhale/Exhale* Graphic Organizer on the right section. On each tab:

✎ Color the lungs blue and the diaphragm red. Open the tabs. Draw a picture of yourself breathing in air. Draw a picture breathing out.
✎✎ Color the lungs blue and the diaphragm red. Open the tabs. Write clue words about inhalation and exhalation. *Inhale air, air to lungs, blood to lungs, get oxygen, give off carbon dioxide, oxygen blood to heart, exhale carbon dioxide.*

✎✎✎ On the Inhale tab, draw red arrows showing oxygen going into the body. On the Exhale tab, draw blue arrows showing carbon dioxide leaving the body. Label the parts of the graphics. Open the tabs. Explain what happens to oxygen and carbon dioxide during inhalation and exhalation.

This completes the *Cardiovascular and Respiratory Systems Shutter Fold.* Prepare a simple oral presentation using your Graphic Organizer.

Experiences, Investigations, and Research

Select one or more of the following activities for individual or group enrichment projects. Allow your students to determine the format in which they would like to report, share, or graphically present what they have discovered. This should be a creative investigation that utilizes your students' strengths.

 1. Research the relationship between smoking and respiratory diseases. Write a report on your findings and share it with two people.

 2. Learn the Heimlich maneuver.

3. Take a First Aid or CPR (Cardio Pulmonary Resuscitation) course.

4. Imagine you are an oxygen molecule traveling through the respiratory system. Describe your journey.

5. Make a poster about good nutrition, exercise, and rest.

6. http://www.howstuffworks.com/lung1.htm

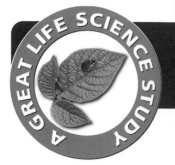
What is the nervous system?

Human Body Concepts:

- The nervous system consists of the brain, spinal cord, and nerves.
- The spinal cord is a bundle of nerves that run through the backbone.
- The central nervous system is made up of the brain and spinal cord.
- The peripheral nervous system is made up of nerves connecting the brain and spinal cord to other body parts.
- Nerves are made of up thousands of neurons.
- The peripheral nervous system consists of the voluntary and involuntary systems.

Vocabulary Words: nervous system   nerves   spinal cord   backbone   *reflex
*CNS (central nervous system)   *PNS (peripheral nervous system)   *neurons   *axon
*dendrite   *cell body   *synapse

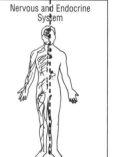

Construct and Read: *Lots of Science Library Book #10.*

Activities:

Nervous System - Graphic Organizer

Focus Skills: labeling
Paper Handouts: 12" x 18" construction paper   8.5" x 11" sheet of paper
    a copy of Graphic 10A - C
Graphic Organizer: Using the 12" x 18" construction paper, make a Shutter Fold. Label it
    Nervous and Endocrine Systems. Glue/copy Graphic 10A on the left side of the
    cover, and Graphic 10B on the right side. Using the 8.5" x 11" paper, make a Hot
    Dog. Keeping the fold on the right side, glue Graphic 10C on the front and label it
    Nervous System. Open the *Nervous and Endocrine Systems Shutter Fold.* Glue the
    Nervous System Graphic Organizer on the left side of the middle section.

✎   Color the brain red; color the spinal cord yellow; color the nerves blue. Open the book.
    On the left side, draw a picture of yourself walking, dreaming, and/or solving problems.

✎✎   Label the parts of the nervous system: *brain, spinal cord, nerves.* Open the book. On
    the left side, write clue words about the nervous system.
    *CNS is brain and spinal cord. PNS has two systems: voluntary –
    nerves of pain, movement; involuntary – breathing, heart
    beating.* Highlight the words *brain* in red, *spinal cord* in
    yellow, and *nerves* in blue.

✎✎✎   Label the parts of the nervous system: *brain, spinal cord,
    nerves.* Open the book. On the left side, define the parts;
    highlight the words *brain* in red, *spinal cord* in yellow, and

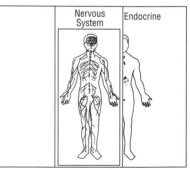

nerves in blue.   Describe the central and peripheral nervous systems. Compare and contrast the voluntary and involuntary nervous systems.

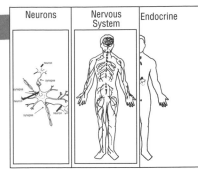

Neurons - Graphic Organizer

Focus Skill: explaining a function
Paper Handouts: 8.5" x 11" sheet of paper   Graphics 10D - E
Graphic Organizer: Make a Hot Dog and, keeping the fold on the
left side, glue/copy Graphic 10D on the cover. Label it
Neurons. Open the Hot Dog. Glue/copy Graphic 10E on the
right side. Open the *Nervous and Endocrine Systems Shutter
Fold*. Glue the *Neuron* Hot Dog on the left section of the
Nervous and Endocrine Systems Shutter Fold. Open the *Neuron* Hot Dog. On the left side:

✎ Draw a cell body, dendrite, and axon.

✎✎ Write clue words about cell body, dendrite, and axon: *cell body - contains nucleus and nerve fibers, dendrite - receives for cell body, axon - sends information from cell body.*

✎✎✎ Describe and explain the functions of cell body, dendrite, and axon.

You will use the *Nervous and Endocrine Systems Shutter Fold* in
Lessons 11 and 22.

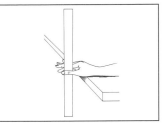

Investigative Loop - Reaction Time

Focus Skill: recording data
Lab Materials: yardstick
Paper Handouts: Lab Book   Lab Record Cards   Lab Graphic 10-1
Graphic Organizer: Glue Lab Graphic 10-1 on the right pocket of the   Lab Book.
Question: How fast/slow is my reaction time? On a Lab Record Card labeled "Lab 10-1," write
the question.
Procedure: Place your hand at the edge of a table. Your partner will hold the yardstick (1-inch
mark on the bottom) just above your hand. When your partner releases the yardstick,
catch it with your thumb and forefinger. Record this number. Do this several times.
Observations: Observe where your hand caught the yardstick. Did you observe any pattern to
your reaction time? Did your reaction time increase or decrease as you continued to
perform the activity? What was the average?
Record the Data: On a Lab Record Card labeled "Lab 10-1," record the number on the yardstick
where your thumb and forefinger caught the yardstick after each catch.
Conclusions: Draw conclusions about your reaction time.
Communicate the Conclusions: On a Lab Record Card labeled "Lab 10-1," write your
conclusions.
Spark Questions: Discuss questions sparked by this lab.
New Loop: Choose one question to investigate further.

Note: A similar Investigative Loop will be completed in Lessons 14 and 17.

Knee-Jerk Reflex

Activity: Ask your partner to sit on a chair and cross his legs comfortably. Quickly and firmly
tap about 3-4 cm below his kneecap with the side of your hand. Note: The lower part
of the leg will swing upward. Trade places with your partner.

Experiences, Investigations, and Research

Select one or more of the following activities for individual or group enrichment projects. Allow your students to determine the format in which they would like to report, share, or graphically present what they have discovered. This should be a creative investigation that utilizes your students' strengths.

1. List/draw activities involving the voluntary and involuntary nervous systems.

2. Drop a dollar bill from a high point and ask your partner to catch it as it flutters to the ground. Trade places. Why do you think this was difficult?

3. Read this sentence: Simple Simon met a pie man going to the fair. Write the sentence quickly on a sheet of paper without dotting the i's or crossing the t's. Describe the difficulty of this assignment.

4. Research and describe how many miles of nerves are found in the human body.

Notes

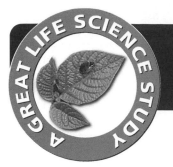
What do we know about the brain?

Human Body Concepts:
- The brain controls all the body's activities.
- The brain consists of the brainstem, cerebellum, and cerebrum.
- The brainstem controls basic body functions such as breathing, heartbeat, and digestion.
- The cerebellum maintains posture, balance, and coordination of body movements.
- The cerebrum consists of the right and left cerebral hemispheres.
- The cortex is the outer layer of the cerebrum and controls processes such as thinking, reasoning, learning, and memory.

Vocabulary Words: brain   right   left   think   memory   *brainstem *cerebellum
*cerebrum   *cortex   *frontal lobe   *temporal lobe

Construct and Read: *Lots of Science Library Book #11.*

Activities:

Parts of the Brain – Graphic Organizer

Focus Skill: labeling and listing
Paper Handouts: 8.5" x 11" sheet of paper   a copy of Graphics 11A - C
Nervous and Endocrine Systems Shutter Fold
Graphic Organizer: Make a 3 Tab Hot Dog with the fold on top. Glue/copy Graphics 11A-C on each tab. Label each tab *Cerebrum, Brainstem,* and *Cerebellum* accordingly. Fold the left tab over the middle tab, and the right tab over the middle. Label the cover *Parts of the Brain.* Open the *Nervous and Endocrine Systems Shutter Fold.* Open the *Nervous System* book. Glue the *Parts of the Brain* on the top left side.

On each tab:
✎ Color the cerebrum gray; color the brainstem red; color the cerebellum blue. Open the tabs. Draw pictures of yourself using your brain.
✎✎ Label the parts of the brain: *cerebrum, brainstem, cerebellum.* Open the tabs. Write clue words about each part of the brain. cerebellum – *keeps balance and coordination of body.* cerebrum – *85% of brain's weight, thinking, reasoning, memory.* brainstem – *communicates to body.*
✎✎✎ Label the parts of the brain: *cerebrum, brainstem, cerebellum.* Open the tabs. List the functions each part helps to perform.

Parts of the Brain		

Brain Lobes – Graphic Organizer

Focus Skill: applying information

Paper Handouts: 8.5" x 11" sheet of paper   a copy of Graphics 11D - G

Graphic Organizer: Fold a Large Question and Answer Book but do not cut the tabs. Label the cover *Brain Lobes*. Open the *Nervous and Endocrine Systems Shutter Fold*. Open the *Nervous System* tab. Glue the Large Question and Answer Book on the bottom left side. Open the Large Question and Answer Book completely. You will see folds or cuts defining four sections. Glue/copy Graphics 11D - G on the top part of each section.

Label the tabs *Frontal Lobe, Parietal Lobe, Occipital Lobe,* and *Temporal Lobe* accordingly.

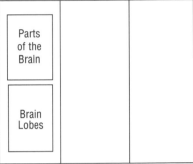

Color the frontal lobe on the *Frontal Lobe* tab; color the parietal lobe on the *Parietal* tab; repeat for the remaining two tabs. Under each graphic:

✎ Draw a picture of yourself performing an activity

✎✎ Write clue words about each lobe. frontal – *voluntary muscles, intelligence & personality.* temporal – *hearing and memory.* parietal – *body awareness senses.* occipital – *vision.*

✎✎✎ Describe the activities in which each lobe is involved.

Investigative Loop – Memory

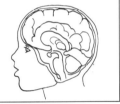

Focus Skill: making observations

Lab Materials: assorted small school and/or household items

Paper Handouts: 8.5" x 11" sheet of paper   Lab Book   new Lab Record Cards   Lab Graphic 11-1

Graphic Organizer: Make a Pocket Book and glue it side-by-side to the existing Lab Book. Glue Graphic 11-1 on the left pocket.

Concept: Memory can improve with practice.

Prediction: On a Lab Record Card labeled "Lab 11-1," predict whether your memory can improve with practice.

Procedure: Place 20 small objects on the table (ex: toothpick, comb, pen, sock, button, etc.) Cover the table with a sheet. Remove the sheet and let your partner view the objects for 30 seconds, then cover it again. Ask your partner to write (or name) as many items as possible. Trade places and ask your partner to select 20 new objects. Complete the activity at least two more times, using new objects each time.

Observations: After the objects are uncovered, write (or name) as many items as you can remember. Make quantitative observations of the number of items remembered after each session. Did your memory improve or get worse? What was the highest number? the lowest number? the average?

Record the Data: After each observation, record the number of objects remembered.

Conclusions: Draw conclusions about what you observed.

Communicate the Conclusions: On a Lab Record Card labeled "Lab 11-1," write your conclusions.

Spark Questions: Discuss questions sparked by this lab.

New Loop: Choose one question and investigate it further. Or, repeat the same procedure but try various techniques to improve memory, such as grouping items together, handling them, naming the items out loud, etc.

Right and Left Brain

Activity Materials: sheet of paper   pen or pencil

Activity: Stand in front of a desk holding a pen in your dominate hand. Place the sheet of paper in front of you. Rotate your right foot in a clockwise motion. While rotating your foot, write a large number 6 on the paper. Were you able to do it? What happened to your right foot? Repeat the procedure with the left foot rotating clockwise while you write the number 6. Repeat the procedure with counterclockwise motions. Which combination was the easiest? Why? **The right side of the body is controlled by the left side of the brain; the left side of the body is controlled by the right side of the brain.**

Experiences, Investigations, and Research

Select one or more of the following activities for individual or group enrichment projects. Allow your students to determine the format in which they would like to report, share, or graphically present what they have discovered. This should be a creative investigation that utilizes your students' strengths.

1. Investigate the size and shape of the human brain. How do lobes increase the brain's surface area? Why is this important?

2. What is a concussion and how does it effect the brain?

3. Compare the walnut-sized brain of a Stegosaurus to the human brain. Is there a relationship between brain size and intelligence?

4. How is a person's IQ measured? Do you think IQ is something that can be accurately measured? Why or why not?

5. Research and compare "right brain" and "left brain" learning styles. Are you right-brained or left-brained?

Notes

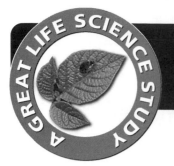

Great Science Adventures

Lesson 12

What do we know about sight?

Human Body Concepts:

- A human eye consists of an iris, pupil, lens, cornea, retina, and optic nerve.
- The retina is the light-sensitive part of the eye which consists of rods and cones.
- Rods work well in dim light; cones work well in bright light.

Vocabulary Words: sight   senses   iris   pupil   lens   focus   image *cornea
*retina   *rods   *cones   *optic nerve

Construct and Read: *Lots of Science Library Book #12.*

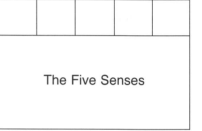

The Five Senses

Activities:

Parts of the Human Eye – Graphic Organizer

Focus Skill: labeling
Paper Handouts: 7 sheets of 8.5" x 11" paper   a copy of Graphics 12A - D
Graphic Organizer: Make a 5 Top Tab Book, see page xiv. Label the cover *The Five Senses.* Glue/copy Graphic 12A on the far left tab. Open the page for that tab. Glue/copy Graphic 12B on the top right side. Label it *Parts of the Human Eye.*

✎ Draw two eyes

✎✎ ✎✎✎ Label the parts of the eye: *pupil, iris, lens, rods, cones*

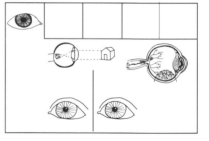

Glue/copy Graphic 12C on the top left side. Label it *How Does the Human Eye See?* Discuss or write a brief description of how human eyes see an object.

Bright Light and Dim Light

Activity: Stand in front of a mirror. Cover your eyes with your hands for about 30 seconds, keeping your eyes open. Remove your hands and immediately look in the mirror. What did you see? Try it again.
Graphic Organizer: Glue/copy Graphic 12D on the bottom left side. Color the iris and, with a black marker, draw the pupil in bright light; draw the pupil in dim light.

You will be adding to this Top Tab Book in Lessons 14-17. This will be referred to as *The Five Senses Top Tab Book.*

Blind Spot

Complete the activity in *Lots of Science Library Book #12*, pages 13 and 14.

What Color Are Your Socks?

Activity Materials: variety of colored socks
Activity: In a dark room, spread the socks out in front of you. Try to find matching pairs of socks. Turn on the light. How well did you do?
Optional: Repeat the procedure using a flashlight with colored cellophane over the light.

Two Eyes are Better than One

Activity Materials: blindfold   ball
Activity: Toss a ball back and forth with your partner. Now, blindfold one eye. Toss the ball again. Was it harder to catch? Why?

Hole in the Hand

Activity Materials: sheet of paper
Activity: Roll up a sheet of paper to make a telescope. Look through the telescope with your right eye. Hold your left hand about 4 inches in front of your left eye. What do you see? **Your hand will appear to have a hole.**

Experiences, Investigations, and Research

Select one or more of the following activities for individual or group enrichment projects. Allow your students to determine the format in which they would like to report, share, or graphically present what they have discovered. This should be a creative investigation that utilizes your students' strengths.

1. Close your eyes and gently place your finger over your eyelid. Very gently move your finger from corner to corner. The curved lump you feel is the cornea.

2. Visit your local butcher, meatpacker, or slaughterhouse and ask for a sheep or beef eye. Examine the eye. Locate the optic nerve. Using a sharp utensil, carefully cut away the tissue covering the eye ball. Cut through the cornea and remove the lens. Locate the iris.

3. http://www.howstuffworks.com/eye.htm

4. Read *Helen Keller: Courage in the Dark* by Johanna Hurwitz.

5. Read *Helen Keller* by Margaret Davidson.

6. Make a poster explaining ways in which a person can protect their vision.

7. Compare and contrast near sighted, far sighted, and perfect vision.

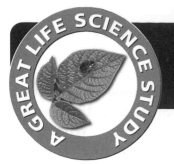

What do we know about perception?

Human Body Concepts:

- Perception is how the brain processes what is seen.
- An optical illusion occurs when two objects produce the same images but are perceived differently.

Vocabulary Words: circle   lines   size   shape   bright   dim   *perception
*constancy   *aftereffect   *optical illusion

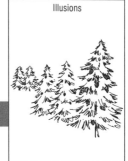

Illusions

Construct and Read: *Lots of Science Library Book #13.*

Activities:

Illusions – Graphic Organizer

Focus Skills: collecting and analyzing data
Paper Handouts: 3 sheets of 8.5" x 11" paper   a copy of Graphics 13A - G
Graphic Organizer: Using the 3 sheets of paper, make a Bound Book. Glue/copy Graphic 13A on the cover and label it *Illusions*. Open the book, skip the page behind the cover and glue Graphic 13B on the next page. Skip the page behind Graphic 13B, and glue Graphic 13C on the next page. Continue with Graphics 13D - 13F. You should have a graphic on every other page.

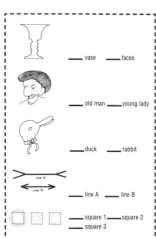

Ask ten people if you can test their perceptual skills. Show them Graphic 13B and ask, "What is the first thing you see in this design?" On 13G, use tally marks to record *vase* or *faces*. For Graphic 13C, ask the same question and record *old man* or *young lady*. For Graphic 13D, ask the same question, and record *duck* or *rabbit*. For Graphic 13E, ask, "Which line is longer?" Be sure to measure the lines to know the correct answer. Record line *A* or *B*. For Graphic 13F, ask, "Which is a perfect square?" Be sure to measure each side to know the correct answer. Record square *1, 2,* or *3*.

You may also write down the age of the person to compare answers by age. You may write down if they are a boy or a girl to compare answers by sex. For this type of data collection you will need a copy of 13G for each person tested. Graph your data, if possible.

Activity Materials: 2 index cards   ruler   black, red, and blue markers

Activity: Draw a 2" x 2" square in the middle of an index card. Draw a 1" x 1" square inside the 2" square. Color the outer square blue and the inner square red. Stare at both squares for at least 30 seconds. Look away at a white wall or a white sheet of paper. What did you see? On the other index card, draw a 3" X in the middle. With your marker, thicken the X so it is about $1/2$" thick. In filtered lighting, stare at the X for at least 30 seconds. Look away at a white wall or a white sheet of paper. What did you see?

Experiences, Investigations, and Research

Select one or more of the following activities for individual or group enrichment projects. Allow your students to determine the format in which they would like to report, share, or graphically present what they have discovered. This should be a creative investigation that utilizes your students' strengths.

1. Design an optical illusion and note how friends and family respond when they view it.

2. Find illusion books from your local library.

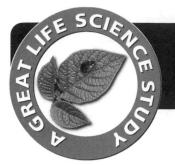

Great Science Adventures

What do we know about hearing?

Human Body Concepts:

- A human ear consists of the outer ear, middle ear, and inner ear.
- The outer ear consists of the auricle, which collects sound waves.
- Sound waves move to the middle ear, which consists of the eardrum, hammer, anvil, and stirrup.
- When sound waves hit the eardrum, it vibrates and passes the vibrations through to the inner ear, which consists of the cochlea.
- Sound waves are changed into electrical signals and sent along the auditory nerve to the brain.

Vocabulary Words: sound   outer ear   middle ear   inner ear   vibrates   deaf

*auricle   *hammer   *anvil   *stirrup   *cochlea   *auditory

Construct and Read: *Lots of Science Library Book #14.*

👁	🧒		

The Five Senses

Activities:

Parts of the Human Ear – Graphic Organizer

Focus Skill: labeling
Paper Handouts: *Five Senses Top Tab Book*   Graphics 14A - D
Graphic Organizer: Glue/copy Graphic 14A on the second tab from the left of the *Five Senses Top Tab Book.* Glue/copy Graphic 14B on the right side of that page. Label it *Parts of the Human Ear.*

✏ Highlight the outer ear pink; middle ear blue; inner ear yellow.

✏✏ Label the parts of the ear: *auricle, ear canal, eardrum, hammer, anvil, stirrup, cochlea, auditory nerve*

✏✏✏ Label the parts of the ear: *auricle, ear canal, tympanic membrane, drum, hammer, anvil, stirrup, malleus, incus, stapes, cochlea, semicircular canals,* and *vestibule.*

How Does the Human Ear Hear?

Glue/copy Graphic 14C on the middle section; glue/copy Graphic 14D on the left side. Label it How *Does the Human Ear Hear?* Draw sound waves from the flute to the ear. Discuss or write how the ear hears the sounds of the flute.

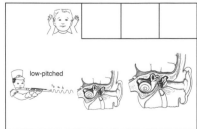

Investigative Loop - Reaction Time with Hearing

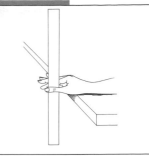

Focus Skill: demonstrating a concept
Lab Materials: yardstick   blindfold
Paper Handouts: Lab Book   Lab Record Cards   Lab Graphic 14-1
Graphic Organizer: Glue Lab Graphic 14-1 on the right pocket of the Lab Book.
Question: What is the reaction time to sounds? Write the question on a Lab Record Card labeled "Lab 14-1."
Procedure: Blindfold yourself. Place your hand on the edge of the table. Your partner will hold the yardstick with the 1-inch mark at the bottom, just above your hand. At the same that your partner releases the yardstick, he/she will say, "Catch." Catch the yardstick with your hand. Do this several times.
Observations: After each catch of the yardstick, observe where your thumb and forefinger caught the yardstick. Did you observe any pattern to your reaction time? What was the average? How did this compare to your reaction time in Lesson 10?
Record the Data: On a Lab Record Card labeled "Lab 14-1," record the number where your thumb and forefinger caught the yardstick for each time it was dropped.
Conclusions: Draw conclusions about what you observed.
Communicate the Conclusions: On a Lab Record Card labeled "Lab 14-1," write your conclusions.
Spark Questions: Discuss questions sparked by this lab.
New Loop: Choose one question to investigate further, or complete the lab with three different people and compare all the results.

Dizzy Water

Activity Materials: cup water
Activity: Fill a cup half full of water. Move the cup in a circular manner to make the water swirl. As the water swirls, place the cup on the table. Observe the movement of the water. What do you see? Compare the movement of the water to why you get dizzy.

Two Ears are Better than One

Activity Materials: radio   blindfold
Activity: Blindfold your partner and turn on the radio. Ask your partner to point to the direction of the radio. Ask your partner to plug one ear. Move the radio to another location and turn it on. Ask your partner to point to the direction of the radio. Trade places. What does this activity demonstrate about hearing with one or both ears?

What Can You Hear?

Activity Materials: blindfold   various objects that make noise, such as: paper, stapler, pencil, scissors, can opener
Activity: Blindfold your partner. Ask your partner to guess what you are doing as you tear a piece of paper, staple paper, cut paper with scissors, use a can opener, etc. Trade places and use other objects. What can you conclude about your sense of hearing?

Experiences, Investigations, and Research

Select one or more of the following activities for individual or group enrichment projects. Allow your students to determine the format in which they would like to report, share, or graphically present what they have discovered. This should be a creative investigation that utilizes your students' strengths.

1. Learn the Sign Language Alphabet.

2. Read a biography on Helen Keller.

3. http://www.howstuffworks.com/hearing4.htm

4. How can loud sounds cause permanent hearing loss?

5. Use ear plugs when talking to a friend. Can you read their lips?

6. Determine if commercials are louder than regular television shows and explain why or why not this occurs.

Notes

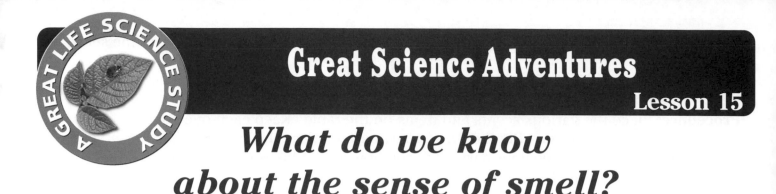

What do we know about the sense of smell?

Human Body Concepts:

- Receptors on the roof of the nasal cavity pick up smells as they enter the nose.
- Nerves connected to these receptors send odor information to the olfactory bulb.
- The olfactory bulb sends signals to the brain.
- Smell is closely linked with the sense of taste.

Vocabulary Words: smell   odors   nose   nostrils   sniffing   *nasal cavity
*smell receptors   *olfactory bulb

Construct and Read: *Lots of Science Library Book #15.*

The Five Senses

Activities:

Parts of the Nose – Graphic Organizer

Focus Skill: labeling
Paper Handouts: *Five Senses Top Tab Book*   Graphics 15A - C
Graphic Organizer: Glue/copy Graphic 15A on the third tab. Glue/copy Graphic 15B on the right side. Label it *Parts of the Nose.*

✎ With a yellow highlighter, draw a line to represent scent entering the nasal cavity.

✎✎ Complete ✎. Label the parts of the nose: *nostrils, nasal cavity, smell receptors, olfactory bulb, olfactory nerve.*

✎✎✎ Label the parts of the nose. Explain how each part benefits the whole nose.

How Does the Human Nose Smell?

Glue/copy Graphic 15C on the left side. Label it *How Does the Human Nose Smell?* Draw lines to represent scent from the bread to the nasal cavity.

Investigative Loop – The Nose Knows

Focus Skill: demonstrating a concept
Lab Materials: ripe banana   peanut butter   blindfold
watch with a second hand   other fruits

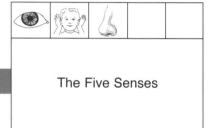

Paper Handouts: 8.5" x 11" sheet of paper   Lab Book
Lab Record Cards   Lab Graphics 15-1
Graphic Organizer: Make a Pocket Book and glue it side-by-side to the Lab Book. Glue Lab Graphic 15-1 on the left pocket.
Question: How quickly can you detect various scents?

Research: Read *Lots of Science Library Book #15* and review what you know about the sense of smell.

Prediction: On a Lab Record Card labeled "Lab 15-1," write how long you think it will take to identify each scent.

Procedure: Place the various scents and items on the table. Keep each one covered in a jar or baggie until needed. Blindfold your partner and place the scents about 10 feet away from him/her. Time your partner to see how long it takes to identify each scent. Repeat the activity with each of the other scents.

Observations: Observe the length of time it took to identify each scent.

Record the Data: On a Lab Record Card labeled "Lab 15-1," write the name of each scent in the order you present them, numbering the scents as you write their names. Record the time it takes for your partner to identify each scent.

Conclusions: Draw conclusions about what you observed, based on the order in which the scents were presented and the type of scent.

Communicate the Conclusions: On a Lab Record Card labeled "Lab 15-1," write your conclusions.

Spark Questions: Discuss questions sparked by this lab.

New Loop: Choose one question to investigate further.

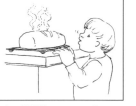

LifeSavers™

Activity Materials: various fruit-flavored Life Savers TM   blindfold

Activity: Blindfold your partner. Give him/her one of the Life Savers TM and ask, "What is the flavor?" Repeat this with several flavors, giving your partner a drink of water between each flavor. Now, with your partner still blindfolded, ask him to plug his/her nose and repeat the activity. Did your partner successfully guess the flavors with the nose unplugged? With it plugged? What does this tell you about smell and taste?

Smell Away

Activity Materials: blindfold   slice of lemon

Activity: Blindfold your partner. Hold a slice of lemon under your partner's nose and ask him to tell you when the lemon has been moved away. Do not move the lemon. What was your partner's reaction? Why?

Experiences, Investigations, and Research

Select one or more of the following activities for individual or group enrichment projects. Allow your students to determine the format in which they would like to report, share, or graphically present what they have discovered. This should be a creative investigation that utilizes your students' strengths.

1. Make a collage using pictures of things that you think smell; good and/or bad.

2. Compare and contrast natural scents and artificial scents.

3. Experiment with solution concentration and dilution. Investigate how much or how little of a scent is needed for detection. For example, find out how many drops of vinegar must be placed in a cup of water for someone to detect its smell. Use various scents. Survey others.

4. Make a list of adjectives that describe smells, such as sweet, flowery, and sour.

5. Prepare a sampling of foods, such as peanut butter, slices of fruits, vinegar, honey, etc. Blindfold your partner and ask him to guess each food. Trade places and use a different group of foods.

6. http://www.howstuffworks.com/framed.htm?parent=question139.htm

7. http://www.sfn.org/briefings/smell.html

Notes

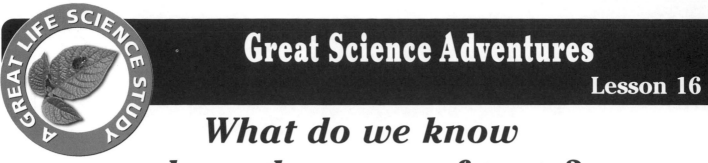

What do we know about the sense of taste?

Human Body Concepts:

- Taste makes eating a pleasurable experience, but it also serves to keep you from eating spoiled food.
- Taste is influenced by smell, food texture, temperature, and appearance.
- The tongue is the human body's main organ for taste.
- Taste buds distinguish four main flavors: sweet, sour, salty, and bitter.

Vocabulary Words: taste   tongue   bumps   sweet   sour   salty   bitter

*taste buds

Construct and Read: *Lots of Science Library Book #16.*

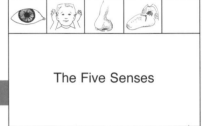

The Five Senses

Activities:

Taste – Graphic Organizer

Focus Skill: labeling
Paper Handouts: *Five Senses Top Tab Book*   Graphics 16A - B
Graphic Organizer: Glue/copy Graphic 16A - B on the fourth tab of the *Five Senses Top Tab Book*. Glue/copy Graphic 16B on the right side. Label it *Tongue*.

✎ Color the taste buds as follows: sweet - red; salty - yellow; sour - blue; bitter - green.

✎✎ Label the taste buds on the tongue: *sweet, salty, sour, bitter*.
   Write clue words about the large and small bumps on the tongue: *helps to grip food*

✎✎✎ Label the taste buds on the tongue: *sweet, salty, sour, bitter, papillae*. Describe papillae and explain their function.

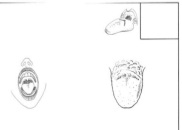

Smell Affects Taste

Glue/copy Graphic 16C on the left side. Label it *Smell Affects Taste*. Discuss or write how smell affects the taste of food.

Investigative Loop – Apple, Potato, or Onion?

Focus Skill: following directions
Lab Materials: apple   potato   onion   blindfold
Paper Handouts: Lab Book   new Lab Record Cards   Lab Graphic 16-1
Graphic Organizer: Glue Lab Graphic 16-1 on the right pocket of the Lab Book.
Question: What affects taste?

Research: Read *Lots of Science Library Book #16* and review what you know about taste.

Prediction: Predict if sight and smell affect taste. Write your prediction on a Lab Record Card labeled "Lab 16-1."

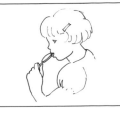

Procedure: Blindfold your partner. Hold a piece of apple in front of your partner's nose as you give him/her a very small piece of potato to chew. Ask him/her to chew it for at least a minute, then swallow. Can he/she identify what was eaten? Give him/her a drink of water after each taste test. Now hold a slice of onion in front of your partner's nose and give him/her a small piece of apple to chew. Can he/she identify what was eaten?

Observations: Observe which item determined your partner's response, the one smelled or the one tasted.

Record the Data: Label a Lab Record Card "Lab 16-1" and record your observations.

Conclusions: Draw conclusions about what affects taste.

Communicate the Conclusions: Label a Lab Record Card "Lab 16-1" and write your conclusions. Sketch a picture of the objects smelled, tasted, and eaten.

Spark Questions: Discuss questions sparked by this lab.

New Loop: Choose one question and investigate it further.

Experiences, Investigations, and Research

Select one or more of the following activities for individual or group enrichment projects. Allow your students to determine the format in which they would like to report, share, or graphically present what they have discovered. This should be a creative investigation that utilizes your students' strengths.

1. Learn several tongue twisters.

2. Why do dentists tell us to brush our tongue as well as our teeth?

3. Keep a food journal for three days. Note which foods you prefer. Are they salty or sweet?

4. Make a chart and list examples of sweet, salty, sour, and bitter foods you see in advertisements. What tastes do you think most people prefer? Why?

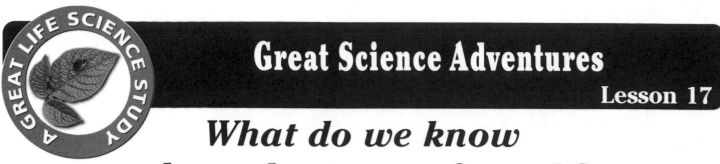

What do we know about the sense of touch?

Human Body Concepts:

- Receptors located under the surface of the skin process sensations of pain, temperature, and pressure.
- Touch receptors are found in the epidermis and dermis.
- Pressure receptors are located in the dermis.

Vocabulary Words: touch   pain   danger   heat   blind   *temperature
*pressure

Construct and Read: *Lots of Science Library Book #17.*

The Five Senses

Activities:

Touch – Graphic Organizer

Focus Skill: labeling
Paper Handouts: *Five Senses Top Tab Book* Graphics 17A - C
Graphic Organizer: Glue/copy Graphic 17A on the last tab. Glue/copy Graphic 17B on the top of the right side of that page.

- ✎ Highlight the light touch receptors pink; the pressure receptors blue; the cold receptors yellow; and pain and heat receptors green.
- ✎✎ Label the following receptors: *light touch receptors, pressure receptors, cold receptors,* and *pain and heat receptors.*
- ✎✎✎ Complete ✎✎✎ Explain the function of these receptors.

Braille

Cut out or copy Graphic 17C. Place the Graphic on a soft surface, such as a cushion. Using the end of a paper clip, punch the dots from the back side. Flip the graphic over and glue it on the left side of the *Touch* tab. Label it *Braille.*

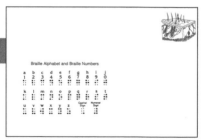

Braille Alphabet and Braille Numbers

This completes your *Five Senses Top Tab Book.* Display your Book and make a simple presentation.

Time with Touch

Focus Skill: recording data

Lab Materials: yardstick   blindfold

Paper Handouts: 8.5" x 11" sheet of paper   Lab Book   Lab Record Cards
   Lab Graphic 17-1

Graphic Organizer: Make a Pocket Book and glue it side-by-side to the Lab Book. Glue Graphic
   17-1 on the left pocket.

Question: How does touch affect your reaction time? Write the question on a Lab Record Card
   labeled "Lab 17-1."

Procedure: Blindfold yourself. Place your hand at the edge of the table. Your partner will hold
   the yardstick (1-inch mark at the bottom) just above your hand. At the same time your
   partner releases the yardstick, he/she will touch your other hand. Catch the yardstick
   with your thumb and forefinger. Do this several times. Trade places with your partner.

Observations: Observe the number mark on the yardstick where your thumb and forefinger
   caught the yardstick each time. Did you observe any pattern to your reaction time?
   What was the average? How did this compare with your reaction time in Lessons 10
   and 14?

Record the Data: On a Lab Record Card labeled "Lab 17-1," record the number on the yardstick
   after each catch.

Conclusions: Draw conclusions about what you observed.

Communicate the Conclusions: On a Lab Record Card labeled "Lab 17-1," write your
   conclusions.

Spark Questions: Discuss questions sparked by this lab.

New Loop: Choose one question to investigate further.

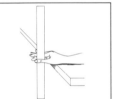

Back Pin Points

Activity Materials: 3 sharpened pencils   tape

Activity: Tape two sharpened pencils together. With the single pencil and the two taped
   pencils, gently prick your partner's back randomly. Ask him/her if he/she felt one or
   two pin points. Trade places with your partner. Were certain areas of the back more
   sensitive than other parts? Compare and contrast your responses and your partner's
   responses.

Pressure Receptors

Activity Materials: bar of soap   2 straight pins   ruler   blindfold

Activity: Place the two straight pins into the bar of soap 3 cm apart.
   IMPORTANT: Place the pointed ends of the straight pins in the bar of soap, exposing
   the heads of the pins. Blindfold your partner. Hold the soap and gently press the
   pinheads on your partner's palm. Ask your partner how many pins were felt. If one
   pin was felt, move the pins 1 cm further apart. If two pins were felt, move the pins 1
   cm closer together. Repeat this procedure until you find the shortest distance at which
   your partner can feel two pins.

   Repeat the same procedure on your partner's forehead, forearm, and back. What part
   of the body has the most receptors? What part has the fewest receptors?

Activity Materials: blindfold   objects such as a cotton ball, a flower, paper, a crumpled ball of aluminum foil, a spoon, sandpaper

Activity: Blindfold your partner. Ask your partner to guess each object by feeling the object with his/her face, arms, or any part of his body except his hands. Trade places with your partner and use a new set of objects to feel. What part of your body helped you the most to identify the objects? What part of your body was least helpful?

Hot and Cold

Activity Materials: blindfold   bowl of hot water   bowl of cold water
bowl of lukewarm water

Activity: Blindfold your partner. Ask your partner to place his/her right hand in the hot water and his/her left hand in the lukewarm water. Ask your partner to describe the temperature of the water in both bowls. Change the positions of the bowls, so that your partner's right hand is placed in the cold water and his/her left hand is in the lukewarm water. Ask him/her to describe the temperature of the water. Trade places. What determined the feeling of warmth or cold? What can you conclude?

Experiences, Investigations, and Research

Select one or more of the following activities for individual or group enrichment projects. Allow your students to determine the format in which they would like to report, share, or graphically present what they have discovered. This should be a creative investigation that utilizes your students' strengths.

 1. Feely Bag – Place a mystery object in a brown paper bag. Ask your students to close their eyes, put their hand inside the bag, and guess the object.

2. Feely Collage – Find materials with various textures and glue them on a poster board. Ex: sandpaper, cotton balls, pieces of fabric, twigs, leaves, feathers, etc.

 3. Learn the Braille alphabet.

4. Your hands are useful in discovering properties of an object. What can you tell from touch? (hot, cold, soft, etc.) What can you tell from sight? (color, brightness, etc.)

5. Coin Bag – Place pennies, nickels, dimes, quarters, and half dollars in a bag. Place your hand in the bag and pull out different coins,

 6. Find a partner. Find an object that you can hold in your hand (without your partner's knowledge). Sit at a desk across from each other. Holding the object under the desk, away from your partner's view, describe the object. Use descriptive words to help your partner guess the object. Trade places.

7. Read *A Picture Book of Louis Braille* by David A. Adler. ✎   ✎✎

8. Read *Louis Braille: The Boy Who Invented Books for the Blind* by Margaret Davidson. ✎✎   ✎✎✎

Notes

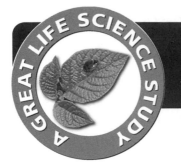
What is the digestive system?

Human Body Concepts:

- Digestion begins in the mouth; teeth chew food and enzymes in saliva help to break down, or digest food.
- The food travels down the esophagus to the stomach.
- Enzymes in the stomach continue the digestive process.
- Most of the absorption occurs in the small intestine through villi.
- Undigested food is excreted.

Vocabulary Words: digestion   hunger   teeth   saliva   stomach   *small intestines
*large intestines   *esophagus   *enzymes   *pancreas   *gallbladder   *villi

Construct and Read: *Lots of Science Library Book #18.*

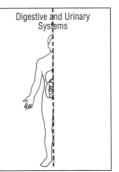

Activities:

Digestive System – Graphic Organizer

Focus Skills: recording information, research
Paper Handouts: 12" x 18" construction paper   8.5" x 11" sheet of paper
    a copy of Graphics 18A - B   *Lots of Science Library Book #18*
Graphic Organizer: Using the 12" x 18" construction paper, make a Shutter Fold. Glue/copy Graphic 18A on the outside of the Shutter Fold, left side. Label it *Digestive and Urinary Systems*. Make a Hot Dog with the 8.5" x 11" paper with the fold on the right side. Glue/copy Graphic 18B on the cover and label it *Digestive System*. Open the Shutter Fold and glue on the middle section. Open the Hot Dog. On the right side:

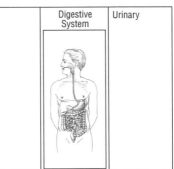

✎   Draw a picture of yourself eating.
✎✎   Sketch a picture of the digestive system, using *Lots of Science Library Book #18* as a resource.
✎✎✎   Complete ✎✎. Explain the digestive process.

Parts of the Digestive System – Graphic Organizer

Focus Skill: explaining a process
Paper Handouts: 8.5" x 11" sheet of paper
    a copy of Graphics 18C - H
Graphic Organizer: Make a Vocabulary Book with 6 tabs. Lay the Vocabulary Book so that the fold is on the left side. Beginning at the top tab, glue/copy Graphics 18C-H in the correct order.

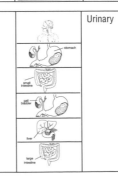

Label them *Esophagus, Stomach, Small Intestine, Pancreas/Gallbladder, Liver,* and *Large Intestine* accordingly.

Under each tab:

✎ Draw each part of the digestive system.

✎✎ Write clue words about each part: esophagus – *lined with mucus; lined with muscles to help push food down; chewed food travels through to stomach through valve at end;* stomach – *wrapped in muscles that churn food with aid of digestive juices; enzymes and acids continue to digest food until it is absorbed;* small intestine – *liquid food travels here and mixes with digestive juices from pancreas and gallbladder; most absorption occurs here into bloodstream through the villi;* pancreas/gallbladder – *digestive juices aid digestion in small intestine;* liver – *largest organ; many jobs; produces bile for digesting fats; filters toxins from blood which is moving back to heart;* large intestine – *remaining food travels here where water is removed to be used by body; undigested food that cannot be used is expelled as waste.*

✎✎✎ Explain the function of each part in the digestive process.

Glue the Vocabulary Book inside the *Digestive System* Hot Dog on the left side.

Digestion Begins in the Mouth – Graphic Organizer

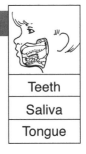

| Teeth |
| Saliva |
| Tongue |

Focus Skill: describing stages in a process

Paper Handouts: 8.5" x 11" sheet of paper   Graphics 18I

Graphic Organizer: Make a Hot Dog and cut on the fold. Using the 2 strips, make a Layered Look Book. Glue/copy Graphic 18I on the cover and label it *Digestion Begins in the Mouth.* Beginning with the top tap, label each *Teeth, Saliva,* and *Tongue.* Color the teeth white, salivary glands yellow, and the tongue pink on Graphic 18I.

✎ Under each tab, draw each part.

✎✎ Open the tabs. Write clue words about each part: *food enters mouth; teeth grind, tongue moves food around; saliva containing enzymes helps break food down.*

✎✎✎ Open the tabs and describe how food is digested in the mouth with the help of teeth, saliva, and tongue.

Glue the Layered Look Book inside the *Digestive and Urinary System Shutter Fold,* on the   left section.

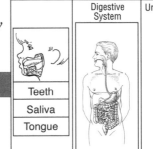

Esophagus

Activity Materials: marble   water   vegetable oil
rubber tubing with hole wide enough for the marble to pass through

Procedure: Moisten the inside of the rubber tubing by running water through it. Put the marble in one end of the tubing. Move the marble through the tube by squeezing the tube behind the marble. Time how long it takes to move the marble through the tubing. Now, moisten the inside of the rubber tubing with oil by placing several drops inside. Flatten the tubing to make sure the entire tube gets coated with oil. (This is a very important step.) Repeat the procedure by squeezing the tube behind the marble. Time how long it takes to move the marble through the tubing.

How long did it take for the marble to pass through the tube moistened with water? How long did it take with oil? What made the difference? Compare the oil to mucus. Compare the squeezing of the rubber tubing to the action in the esophagus.

Note: Follow these directions carefully to avoid choking.
Activity Materials: any food
Procedure: Stand up and bend forward, touching the floor with your hands. Chew a little piece of food and swallow. Did the food travel down the esophagus even though you were upside down? Why? **The walls of the esophagus are lined with muscles that expand and contract to move food through. This process is called peristalsis.**

Cracker to Sugar

Activity Materials: unsalted, unsweetened crackers
Procedure: Chew a piece of cracker but do not swallow it. Describe the taste of the cracker. Bland? Continue chewing for about two minutes. Again, describe the taste of the cracker. What mixed with the cracker as you chewed? **Saliva** How did the saliva help the digestion process? **Saliva wets the food and begins to break it down into smaller pieces before swallowing.** Do you think it is good to chew your food well? **Yes** Why? **The food can be more easily digested in the stomach.**

Experiences, Investigations, and Research

Select one or more of the following activities for individual or group enrichment projects. Allow your students to determine the format in which they would like to report, share, or graphically present what they have discovered. This should be a creative investigation that utilizes your students' strengths.

 1. What is the cause and effect of acid reflux?

 2. Pour a cola drink in a clear glass, add several antacid tablets, and observe what happens.

 3. Compare and contrast the shape, size, and length of the large and small intestines.

4. Do you think the stomach can expand and shrink? Why or why not?

5. Gallbladder surgery is common. How can a person live without a gallbladder?

Notes

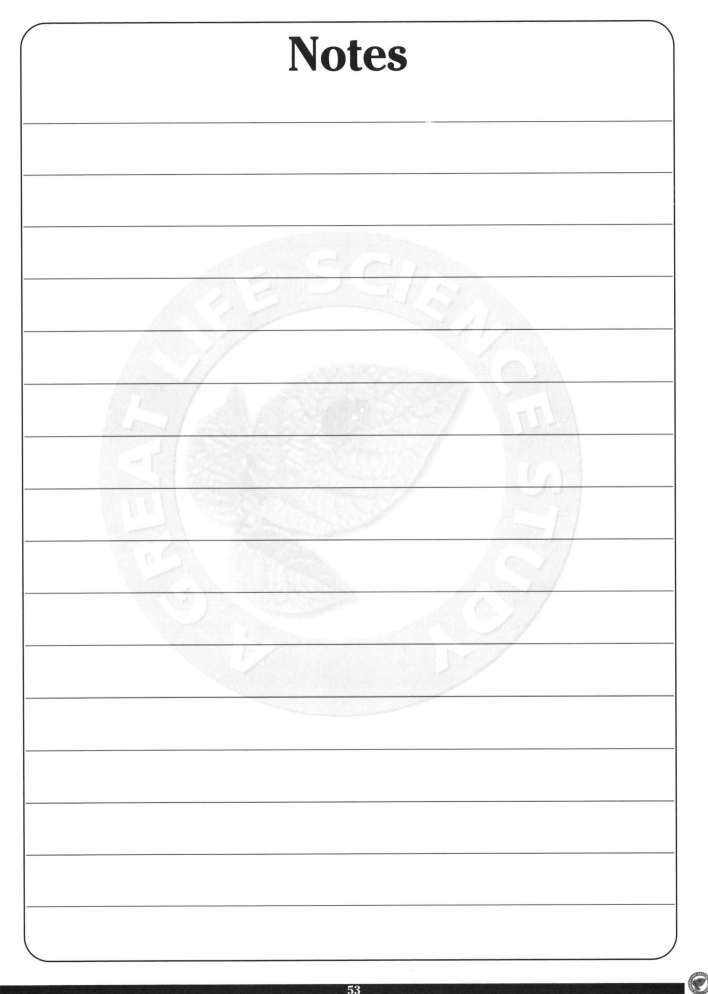

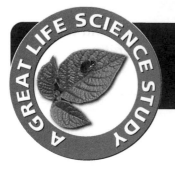
What is the urinary system?

Human Body Concepts:

- The urinary system consists of two kidneys, two ureters, a bladder, and urethra.

Vocabulary Words: filters   cleaned   returned   *kidney   *ureter   *bladder
*urethra   *bile   *liver

Construct and Read: *Lots of Science Library Book #19.*

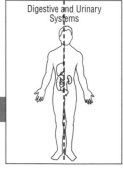

Activities:

Urinary System – Graphic Organizer

Focus Skill: sequencing a process
Paper Handouts: 8.5" x 11" sheet of paper   a copy of Graphics 19A - B
Digestive and Urinary Systems Shutter Fold
Graphic Organizer: Glue/copy Graphic 19A on right side of the Shutter Fold.   Make a Hot Dog
with the 8.5" x 11" paper. With the fold on the left side, glue/copy Graphic 19B on the
cover.   Title it *Urinary System.*

✎   On the cover, use a yellow highlighter to trace the urinary system. Inside, on the left,
draw a glass of your favorite drink.

✎✎   On the left hand side, write clue words about the urinary system: *two kidneys, two
ureters, a bladder, and a urethra; kidneys filter waste products
from the blood; urine goes through the ureters into the bladder;
bladder stores urine.*

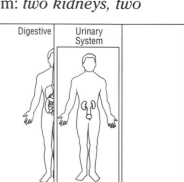

✎✎✎   On the left side, explain the functions of the urinary system.

Parts of the Urinary System – Graphic Organizer

Focus Skill: describing parts of a system
Paper Handouts: 2 sheets of 8.5" x 11"   Graphic 19C-E
Graphic Organizer: Make a Hot Dog and cut on the fold. Make a
Layered Look Book with the two pieces of paper, making 1 1/2 inch tabs. Label the top
tab *Parts of the Urinary System.* Lay the Layered Look Book flat. Cut on the dotted lines
of Graphic 19C and glue each part to the correct tab. Color the kidneys red, ureters
orange, and the bladder yellow. Open the tabs:

✎   On each tab, above the graphic, write *kidneys, ureter,* and *bladder* with corresponding
colored marker.

✎✎   Complete ✎. Write clue words about each part: kidneys – *two, right and left,
located above waist on each side of spine; reddish, bean-shaped organ the size of a bar
of soap; consists of more than a million microscopic filtering units; blood is*

continuously filtered to eliminate waste. ureter – *urine travels through right and left ureters into bladder.* bladder – *stores urine until it is eliminated through urethra.*

✐✐✐ Complete ✐. Explain the function of each component in the urinary system.

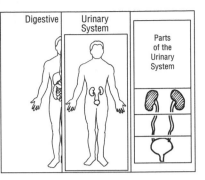

Working with Filters

Activity Materials: bottle   funnel   2 cone-shaped coffee filters
    sugar   water   food coloring   sand

Activity: Fit a piece of filter paper into a funnel. Place the funnel in a bottle. Dissolve some sugar in ¹/₄ cup (120 ml) of water and pour it into the funnel. Does the liquid that drips into the bottle taste sweet? Mix water, food coloring, and sand. Pour it through another filter. What kinds of particles stay on the filter and what kinds go through it?

Experiences, Investigations, and Research

Select one or more of the following activities for individual or group enrichment projects. Allow your students to determine the format in which they would like to report, share, or graphically present what they have discovered. This should be a creative investigation that utilizes your students' strengths.

 1. Research the procedure followed by a medical professional during a urinalysis.

 2. Find out why people who work hard or are very active during hot weather need to drink more liquids. How does salt affect their bodies?

 3. Research kidney dialysis and report on how it works.

 4. Visit your local butcher and ask him for a lamb kidney. (A lamb's kidney is similar to a human's in shape and size.) Slice the kidney lengthwise. Locate the renal vein and artery and nephrons.

5. http://www.howstuffworks.com/kidney7.htm

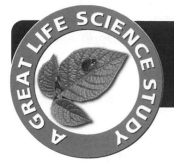
What is the lymphatic system?

Human Body Concepts:

- The lymphatic system is made up of lymph, lymphatic vessels and tissues, and red bone marrow.
- Lymph is a watery fluid that flows through the lymphatic vessels.
- The lymphatic system drains excess fluid from tissues and defends against disease.

Vocabulary Words: drains   defends   carries   attack   *lymph   *lymph node
*lymph duct   *lymphocytes

Construct and Read: *Lots of Science Library Book #20.*

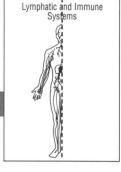

Lymphatic and Immune Systems

Activities:

Lymphatic System – Graphic Organizer

Focus Skill: explaining a process

Paper Handouts: 12" x 18" construction paper   8.5" x 11" sheet of paper
a copy of Graphics 20A - B

Graphic Organizer: Using the 12" x 18" construction paper, make a Shutter Fold Book. Glue/copy Graphics 20A on the left side of the front. Label it *Lymphatic and Immune Systems*. Make a Hot Dog with the 8.5" x 11" paper. With the fold on the right side, glue/copy Graphic 20B on the cover. Title it *Lymphatic System*. Inside, on the leftside: Glue it inside the Shutter Fold, on the left middle section.

✎ Draw the lymphatic System.

✎✎ Write clue words about the functions of the lymphatic system: *made of lymph, lymphatic vessels, tissues, and red bone marrow; drains excess fluid from tissues; helps defend against disease; transports vital vitamins and lipids; lymph carries white blood cells and excess fluid back to blood; lymphatic vessels join together to form larger lymphatic ducts; lymph nodes are bean-shaped and located throughout the body; lymph nodes are where germs are destroyed; two types of white blood cells in lymph node.*

✎✎✎ Explain the functions of the lymphatic system: drains, defends, and transports.

Lymph Node – Graphic Organizer

Focus Skill: describing

Paper Handouts: 8.5" x 11" sheet of paper
a copy of Graphics 20C - D

Graphic Organizer: Make a 2 Tab Hot Dog, with the fold on the left side. Glue/copy Graphic 20C on the top and label it *Lymph*

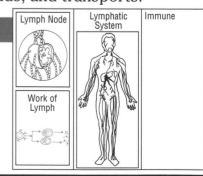

Lymph Node   Lymphatic System   Immune

Work of Lymph

Node. Glue/copy Graphic 20D on the bottom and label it *Work of Lymph.* Open each tab. Under each tab:

✎ Draw a picture of a lymph node and work of the lymph.

✎✎ Write clue words about lymph nodes and work of the lymph: *bean-shaped lymph nodes located throughout body and abundant in neck, armpit, and groin; lymph passes through lymph nodes where germs are destroyed; swollen lymph nodes indicate infection; inside lymph node are macrophages and lymphocytes, which filter lymph that flows through lymph node; macrophages attack and destroy bacteria, viruses, cancer cells, and other harmful agents; lymphocytes release antibodies that locate and destroy specific germs.*

✎✎✎ Describe a lymph node. Explain how lymph travels and its function.
Glue it inside the Shutter Fold, on the far left side.

Experiences, Investigations, and Research

Select one or more of the following activities for individual or group enrichment projects. Allow your students to determine the format in which they would like to report, share, or graphically present what they have discovered. This should be a creative investigation that utilizes your students' strengths.

1. http://www.howstuffworks.com/immune-system4.htm

2. Research leukemia. How does it effect the human body? What are treatments for the disease?

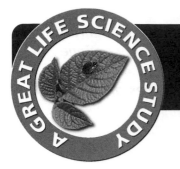

Great Science Adventures

What is the immune system?

Human Body Concepts:

- The immune system defends the human body against infection. It consists mainly of cells in the blood and lymphatic system.
- The immune system depends on lymphocytes to recognize germs and produce antibodies.

Vocabulary Words: immune   germs   disease   *phagocytes *antibodies   *antigen *vaccine

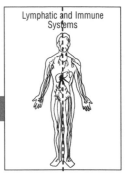

Construct and Read: *Lots of Science Library Book #21.*

Activities:

Immune System – Graphic Organizer

Focus Skills: describing a process
Paper Handouts: 8.5" x 11" sheet of paper   a copy of Graphic 21A - B
Lymphatic and Immune Systems Shutter Fold
Graphic Organizer: Glue/copy Graphic 21A on right side of the Shutter Fold. Make a Hot Dog with the 8.5" x 11" paper. Glue Graphic 21B on the cover. Title it *Immune System*. Open the Shutter Fold and glue the Immune System on the right middle section. Open the Hot Dog:

✎ Draw the immune system battling disease.

✎✎ Write clue words about the immune system: *defends body against infection; consists of cells in blood and lymphatic system; T cells and B cells attack germs; B cells produce antibodies that attach to antigens; when B cell finds antigen, it attaches to it and starts dividing*

✎✎✎ Explain how the immune system functions in the body.

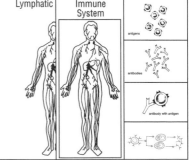

Fighting Germs

Focus Skill: recalling information
Paper Handouts: 8.5" x 11" sheet of paper
a copy of Graphics 21C - F
Graphic Organizer: Make a Hot Dog 4 Tab Book. With the fold on the right side, glue it inside the Shutter Fold on the far right side. Glue/copy Graphics 21C - F on the tabs. Label the tabs *Antigen, Antibodies, Immune, and Vaccine* accordingly. Open the tabs.

✎ Draw a picture of each graphic.

✎✎ Write clue words under each tab: lymphocytes – *recognize a certain antigen, just as a key fits a lock; lymphatic system depends on lymphocytes to recognize germs and produce antibodies.* plasma cells – *when enough B cells are available to fight germs, most of them divide and become plasma cells.* memory cells – *B cells that continue dividing; they remember antigen so that it can attack with needed antibodies if future invasion occurs,* vaccine - *altered form of germ enters body and antibodies are created fro the germ.*

✎✎✎ Explain each part of the immune system.

Experiences, Investigations, and Research

Select one or more of the following activities for individual or group enrichment projects. Allow your students to determine the format in which they would like to report, share, or graphically present what they have discovered. This should be a creative investigation that utilizes your students' strengths.

 1. Research the life of Edward Jenner, Louis Pasteur, Jonas Salk, or Albert Sabin.

2. Research disease prevention and treatment.

3. Choose one person whose studies have helped to advance disease prevention and treatment. Make a poster displaying the contribution of this person.

 4. Find keys to doors, locks, suitcases, etc. Try each key in a lock. Explain how this relates to antigens and antibodies?

5. http://www.howstuffworks.com/immune-system1.htm

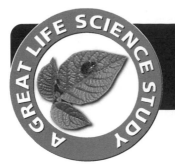

What is the endocrine system?

Human Body Concepts:

- The endocrine system consists of several glands and organs: pituitary, hypothalamus, thyroid, parathyroid, thymus, pancreas, adrenal, ovaries in women and testes in men.
- Endocrine glands produce hormones essential for growth and sexual development.
- The hypothalamus links the endocrine system with the nervous system.

Vocabulary Words: endocrine   messengers   *hypothalamus
*endocrine glands   *hormones   *pituitary glands

Construct and Read: *Lots of Science Library Book #22.*

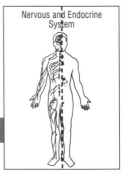

Activities:

Endocrine System – Graphic Organizer

Focus Skills: recalling information

Paper Handouts: 2 sheets of 8.5" x 11" paper   a copy of Graphics 22A - I
    Nervous and Endocrine Systems Shutter Fold from Lesson 10

Graphic Organizer: Make a Hot Dog from one 8.5" x 11" sheet of paper. Glue/copy Graphic 22B on the cover and title it *Endocrine System*. Make a Hot Dog Shutter Fold. Cut both sides into 4 tabs. Glue/copy Graphics B - I on each tab. Under the tab:

✎ Draw a picture of each gland.

✎✎ Write clue words about the function of each gland: pituitary - *controls other hormone producing glands, produces growth hormones, controls kidneys and blood pressure,* hypothalamus - *links endocrine and nervous systems,* thymus - *helps develop antibodies,* adrenal - *increase heart rate, blood flow, sugar levels in times of stress, regulates fluid and mineral balance, and kidneys,* thyroid - *controls energy levels,* parathyroid - *helps control the body's use of calcium,* pancreas - *produces digestive juices, insulin, and allows the liver to store sugar,* sex glands - *produces hormones for the development of male and female characteristics.*

✎✎✎ Explain the function of each gland.
Glue the *Endocrine System* Hot Dog inside the System Shutter Fold, on the middle right. Glue the Hot Dog Shutter Fold on the far right section

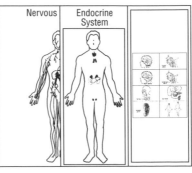

Experiences, Investigations, and Research

Select one or more of the following activities for individual or group enrichment projects. Allow your students to determine the format in which they would like to report, share, or graphically present what they have discovered. This should be a creative investigation that utilizes your students' strengths.

 1. Research adrenaline in the human body. How does it effect the body and why?

 2. Research giant human beings. What type of chemical imbalance causes such growth in certain people?

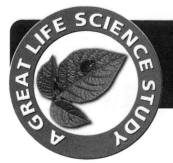

What are the reproductive systems?

Human Body Concepts:

- The reproductive system does not become active until puberty.
- When a sperm and an egg (ova) join, a new life begins.
- A woman's reproductive system consists of ovaries, fallopian tubes, uterus, and vagina.
- A man's reproductive system consists of penis, testes, and urethra.
- Fertilization occurs when a sperm reaches an egg and they fuse forming a zygote.
- The fertilized egg begins to divide and continues to grow and develop.

Vocabulary Words: reproduction   baby   born   male   female   *ovaries
*fallopian tubes   *uterus   *fertilization

Construct and Read: *Lots of Science Library Book #23.*

Reproductive System
and New Life

Activities:

Reproductive System – Graphic Organizer

Focus Skill: describing
Paper Handouts: 12" x 18" construction paper   2 sheets of 8.5" x 11" paper
   a copy of Graphics 23A - F
Graphic Organizer: Using the 12" x 18" construction paper, make a Shutter Fold. Glue Graphic 23A-B on the front of the Shutter Fold. Label it *Reproductive System and New Life*. Make a 2 Tab Hot Dog with the fold on the right side. Glue Graphic 23C on the top tab and title it *Male Reproductive System*. Glue Graphic 23D on the bottom tab and title it *Sperm*. Open the tabs.

✎   Draw a picture of a man.

✎✎   Under each tab, write clue words about the male reproductive system and sperm: *consists of penis, testes, urethra; at puberty two testes produce and store sperm; sperm duct runs from testes to penis through urethra.* sperm: *sperm is much smaller than egg: about .002 inches (.05 mm) long; sperm are flat, with oval head and tail that whips from side to side to move forward; streamlined to making moving through liquids easier.*

✎✎✎   Name and describe the parts of the male reproductive system. Repeat with the sperm tab.

Make another 2 Tab Hot Dog Large Book. Keeping the fold on the left side, glue/copy Graphics 23E - F on the tabs. Label them *Female Reproductive System* and *Egg (Ova)*. Open the tabs and repeat the preceding procedure.

..   Under each tab, write clue words about the female reproduction system and egg: consists of two ovaries, two fallopian tubes, a uterus, and a vagina. egg: *once a month,*

an ovary releases an egg, it travels through fallopian tube to uterus, if it is not fertilized by sperm it moves out of the body.
Glue the Hot Dog 2 Tab Books in the Reproductive System and New Life Shutter Fold, on the middle section, the appropriate side.

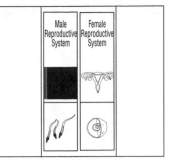

Experiences, Investigations, and Research

Select one or more of the following activities for individual or group enrichment projects. Allow your students to determine the format in which they would like to report, share, or graphically present what they have discovered. This should be a creative investigation that utilizes your students' strengths.

1. Describe and/or sketch the development of a human fetus from fertilization to birth.

2. Research gestation periods of different animal and report your findings by making a chart.

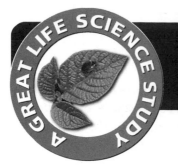
What do we know about new life?

Human Body Concepts:

- The center of every cell is a nucleus, and within each nucleus are stringlike structures called chromosomes.
- An egg contains one female or X-chromosome.
- A sperm contains either one X or one Y-chromosome.
- Each chromosome consists of genes.
- A gene is made up of DNA, the molecules that carry hereditary information.
- During fertilization, the sperm and egg fuse together, resulting in 46 chromosomes.

Vocabulary Words: join   cell division   twins   *DNA (deoxyribonucleic acid)
*chromosomes   *genes   *placenta   *umbilical cord   *amniotic sac   *amniotic fluid

Construct and Read: *Lots of Science Library Book #24.*

Activities:

New Life – Graphic Organizer

Focus Skill: explaining a process
Paper Handouts: 8.5" x 11" sheet of paper   a copy of Graphics 24A - B
Reproductive Systems and New Life Shutter Fold
Graphic Organizer: Make a 2 Tab Hot Dog with the fold on the right side. Glue/copy Graphics 24A-B on the tabs. Open the tabs.

✎ Under each tab, draw a boy and a girl accordingly.

✎✎ Complete ✎. Write clue words about the how a baby's sex is determined under the correct tab. *sperm and egg contain 23 chromosomes; during fertilization, sperm and egg fuse together, resulting in 46 chromosomes; if sperm contains X-chromosome, baby will have two X-chromosomes and be a girl; if sperm contains Y-chromosome, baby will have an X and a Y chromosome and will be a boy.*

✎✎✎ Define chromosomes and genes. Explain the determining factors of a baby's sex. Glue on the left side, inside the *Reproductive Systems and New Life Shutter Fold*

New Life – Graphic Organizer

Focus Skill: describing a process
Paper Handouts: 3 sheets of 8.5" x 11" paper   a copy of Graphics 24C - L
Graphic Organizer: Stack the 3 sheets of paper together and make a Hot Dog. Cut on the folds. Using the 6 strips of paper, make a Layered Look Book with 1-inch tabs. Beginning at the cover, label them: *New Life, Conception, 8 weeks, 12 weeks, 16 weeks, 20 weeks, 24 weeks, Birth, Twins, DNA, Me.* Glue the correct graphic under each tab.

- Draw a picture for each tab in your book. On the last tab, draw a picture of you when you were a baby.

- New Life Cover. Conception – *egg and sperm join in fallopian tube and settle in the uterus, cells divide and grow.* 8 Weeks – *arms and legs are visible, fingers, toes, eyes and ears are developing.* 12 Weeks – *3 inches long, sex organs appear.* 16 Weeks – *8-10 inches long, very active, has finger prints.* 20 Weeks – *12-14 inches long, hears sounds, and weighs about 1 pounds.* 24 Weeks – *eyes are formed, taste buds developed, can inhale, exhale and cry.* 38 Weeks – *ready to be born.* Birth – *about 20 inches and 7-8 pounds.* Twins – *identical, come from same sperm and egg, look exactly alike; fraternal, come from different sperm and egg but are born at the same time.* DNA – *molecules that carry hereditary information, like hair, eye color, skin tone, size and more.* Me – *write information about your birth.*

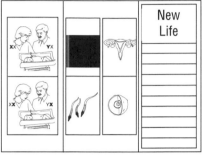

- List information about each stage in new life. On the last tab, interview your parents and write about your time of gestation, birth and early days. Glue on the right side inside the *Reproduction Systems and New Life Shutter Fold.*

Experiences, Investigations, and Research

Select one or more of the following activities for individual or group enrichment projects. Allow your students to determine the format in which they would like to report, share, or graphically present what they have discovered. This should be a creative investigation that utilizes your students' strengths.

1. Research the life of Gregor Mendel and his contributions to science.

2. Discover why DNA is important in police work.

3. http://www.howstuffworks.com/dna-evidence1.htm

4. http://www.howstuffworks.com/framed.htm?parent=link146.htm

5. http://vector.cshl.org/dnaftb/index.html

Notes

Lots of Science Library Books

Each *Lots of Science Library Book* is made up of 16 inside pages, plus a front and back cover. All the covers to the *Lots of Science Library Books* are located at the front of this section. The covers are followed by the inside pages of the books.

How to Photocopy the *Lots of Science Library Books*

As part of their *Great Science Adventure,* your students will create *Lots of Science Library Books.* The *Lots of Science Library Books* are provided as consumable pages which may be cut out of the *Great Science Adventures* book at the line on the top of each page. If, however, you wish to make photocopies for your students, you can do so by following the instructions below.

To photocopy the inside pages of the *Lots Of Science Library Books:*

1. Note that there is a "Star" above the line at the top of each *LSLB* sheet.

2. Locate the *LSLB* sheet that has a Star on it above page 16. Position this sheet on the glass of your photocopier so the side of the sheet which contains page 16 is facing down, and the Star above page 16 is in the left corner closest to you. Photocopy the page.

3. Turn the *LSLB* sheet over so that the side of the *LSLB* sheet containing page 6 is now face down. Position the sheet so the Star above page 6 is again in the left corner closest to you.

4. Insert the previously photocopied paper into the copier again, inserting it face down, with the Star at the end of the sheet that enters the copier last. Photocopy the page.

5. Repeat steps 1 through 4, above, for each *LSLB* sheet.

To photocopy the covers of the *Lots of Science Library Books:*

1. Insert "Cover Sheet A" in the photocopier with a Star positioned in the left corner closest to you, facing down. Photocopy the page.

2. Turn "Cover Sheet A" over so that the side you just photocopied is now facing you. Position the sheet so the Star is again in the left corner closest to you, facing down.

3. Insert the previously photocopied paper into the copier again, inserting it face down, with the Star entering the copier last. Photocopy the page.

4. Repeat steps 1 through 3, above, for "Cover Sheets" B, C, D, E, and F.

How to assemble the *Lots of Science Library Books*

Once you have made the photocopies or cut the consumable pages out of this book, you are ready to assemble your *Lots of Science Library Books*. To do so, follow these instructions:

1. Cut each sheet, both covers and inside pages, on the solid lines.

2. Lay the inside pages on top of one another in this order: pages 2 and 15, pages 4 and 13, pages 6 and 11, pages 8 and 9.

3. Fold the stacked pages on the dotted line, with pages 8 and 9 facing each other.

4. Turn the pages over so that pages 1 and 16 are on top.

5. Place the appropriate cover pages on top of the inside pages, with the front cover facing up.

6. Staple on the dotted line in two places.

You now have completed *Lots of Science Library Books*.

What do we know about the skin?

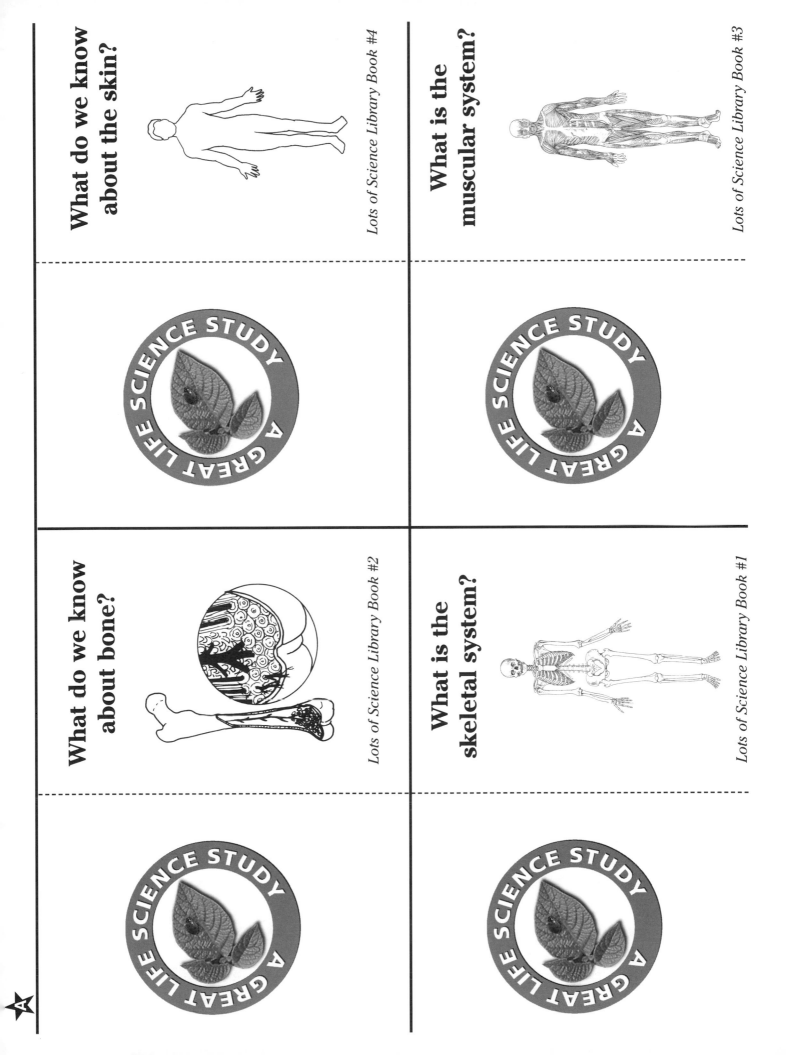

Lots of Science Library Book #4

What is the muscular system?

Lots of Science Library Book #3

SCIENCE STUDY
A GREAT LIFE

SCIENCE STUDY
A GREAT LIFE

What do we know about bone?

Lots of Science Library Book #2

What is the skeletal system?

Lots of Science Library Book #1

SCIENCE STUDY
A GREAT LIFE

SCIENCE STUDY
A GREAT LIFE

skin
epidermis
dermis

* integumentary
* keratin
* melanin
* subcutaneous

Explain the four main
functions of the skin.

What makes up the
integumentary system?

---

bones
calcium

* cartilage
* compact bone
* spongy bone
* red bone marrow
* fracture

Describe the three main
layers of bone.

Where is cartilage located
in your body?

---

muscles
pairs
contracts
oxygen

* ligaments
* involuntary
* voluntary

Describe the three types
of muscles.

---

body
cells
skeleton
joints

* systems
* tissues
* organs
* hinge
* ball-and-socket

Explain the four functions
of the skeleton.

Describe the two main
types of moveable joints.

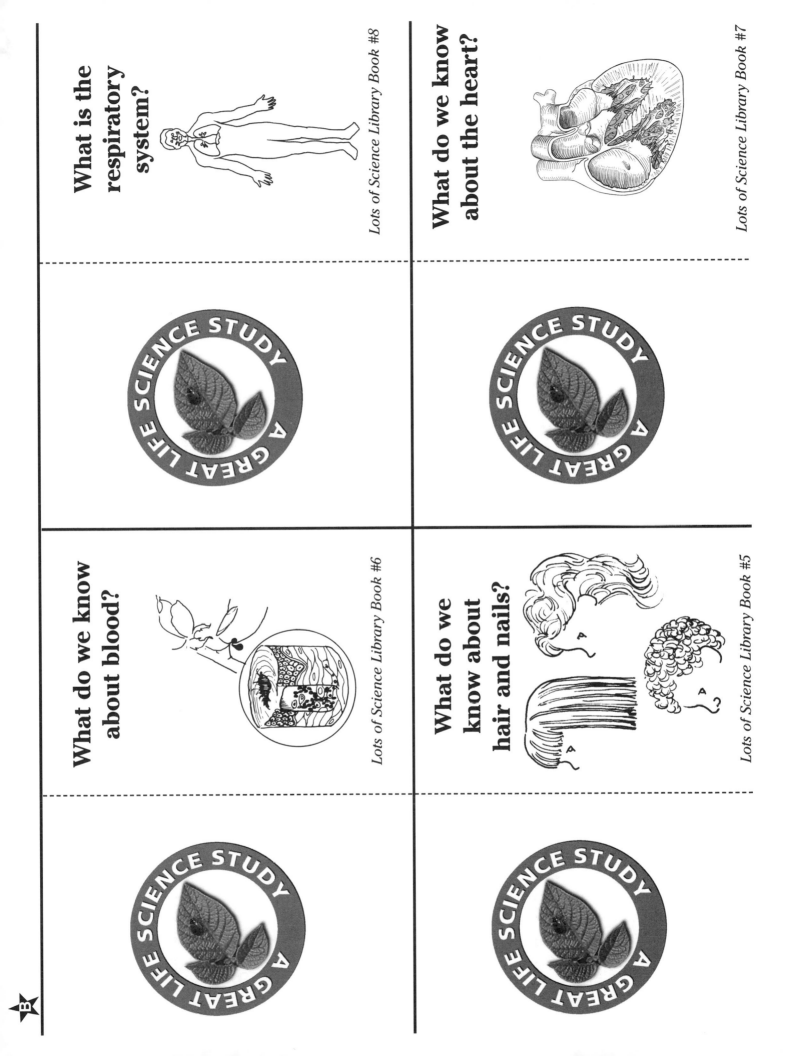

What is the respiratory system?

Lots of Science Library Book #8

What do we know about the heart?

Lots of Science Library Book #7

SCIENCE STUDY
A GREAT LIFE

SCIENCE STUDY
A GREAT LIFE

What do we know about blood?

Lots of Science Library Book #6

What do we know about hair and nails?

Lots of Science Library Book #5

SCIENCE STUDY
A GREAT LIFE

SCIENCE STUDY
A GREAT LIFE

B

B

air
breathe
lungs

* respiratory
* trachea
* lobes
* air sacs
* bronchi

Explain how the respiratory system works in the human body.

blood
clot
carbon dioxide

* cardiovascular
* plasma
* platelets
* hemoglobin

Explain the three main functions of the blood.

Describe the three parts of the blood.

heart
pump
arteries
veins
pulse
circulate

* blood vessels
* capillaries
* aorta
* valves
* atrium
* ventricle

Explain the imortance of the heart to the life of the body.

Compare and contrast the veins and the arteries.

hair
nails
curly
wavy
straight
round
oval
flat

* hair follicle
* nail plate

Explain why some hair is straight and some hair is curly.

Describe how fingernails grow and why it does not hurt to cut them.

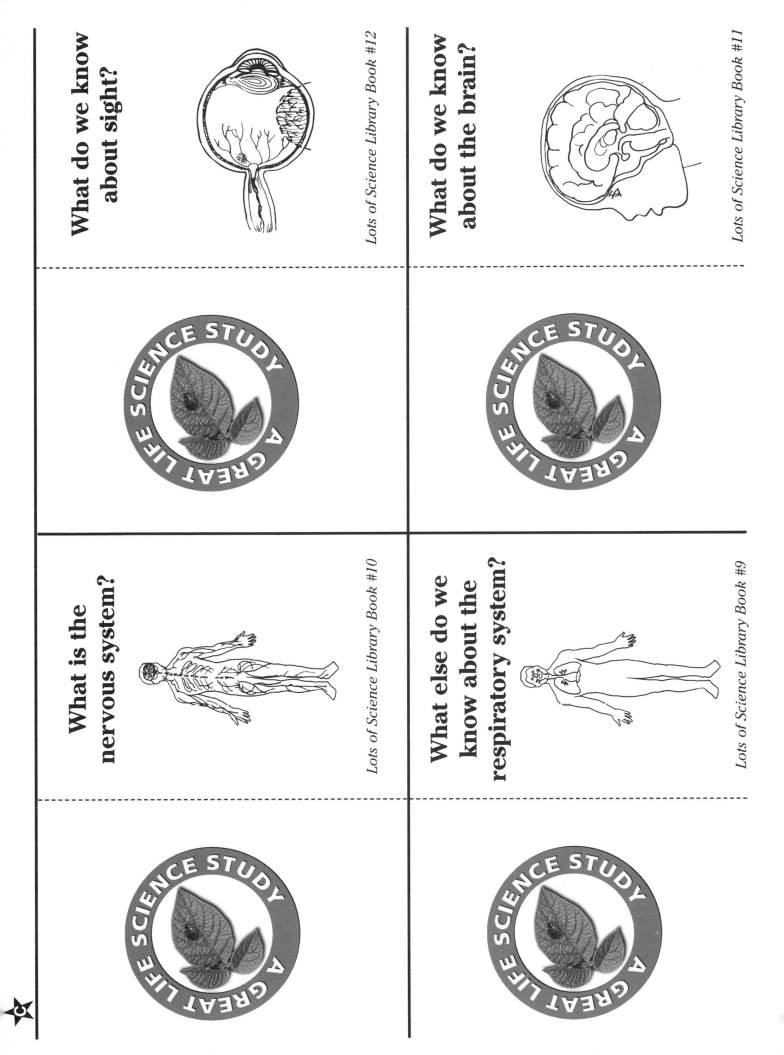

What do we know about sight?

Lots of Science Library Book #12

What do we know about the brain?

Lots of Science Library Book #11

SCIENCE STUDY
A GREAT LIFE

SCIENCE STUDY
A GREAT LIFE

What is the nervous system?

Lots of Science Library Book #10

What else do we know about the respiratory system?

Lots of Science Library Book #9

SCIENCE STUDY
A GREAT LIFE

SCIENCE STUDY
A GREAT LIFE

sight
senses
iris
pupil
lens
focus
image
* cornea
* retina
* rods
* cones
* optic nerve

brain
right
left
think
memory
* brainstem
* cerebellum
* cerebrum
* cortex
* frontal lobe
* temporal lobe

Explain how the human
eye sees an object.

Describe the three parts
of the brain.

nervous system
nerves
spinal cord
backbone
* reflex
* CNS
* PNS
* neurons
* axon
* dendrite
* cell body
* synapse

inhale
exhale
waste
remove
energy
rest
* gas exchange
* diaphragm

Explain the nervous system.

Compare and contrast
voluntary and involuntary
systems.

Explain how the lungs
and heart work together
in gas exchange.

What do we know about the sense of taste?

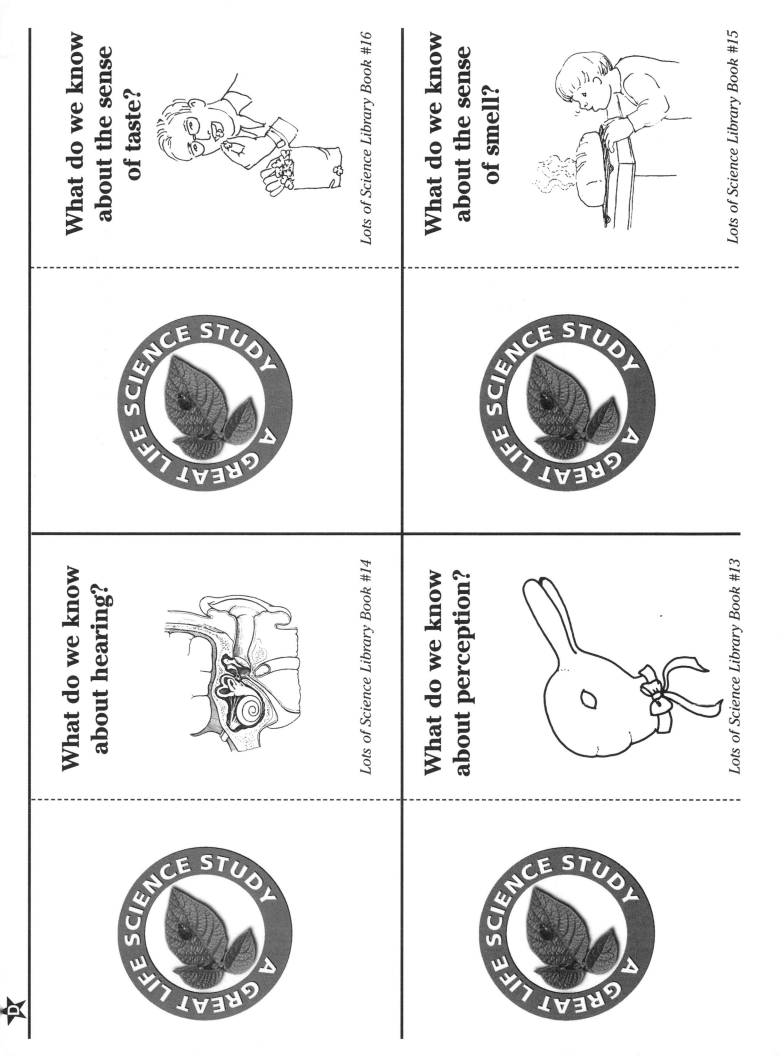

Lots of Science Library Book #16

What do we know about the sense of smell?

Lots of Science Library Book #15

What do we know about hearing?

Lots of Science Library Book #14

What do we know about perception?

Lots of Science Library Book #13

SCIENCE STUDY
A GREAT LIFE

D

taste
tongue
bumps
sweet
sour
salty
bitter

* taste buds

smell
odors
nose
nostrils
sniffing

* nasal cavity
* smell receptors
* olfactory bulb

Explain how the tongue
tastes different foods.

Explain how the nose
smells different scents.

---

sound
outer ear
middle ear
inner ear
vibrates
deaf

* auricle
* hammer
* anvil
* stirrup
* cochlea
* auditory

circle
lines
size
shape
bright
dim

* perception
* constancy
* aftereffect
* optical illusion

Explain how the human
ear hears sound.

Explain the difference
between seeing and
perception.

What is the lymphatic system?

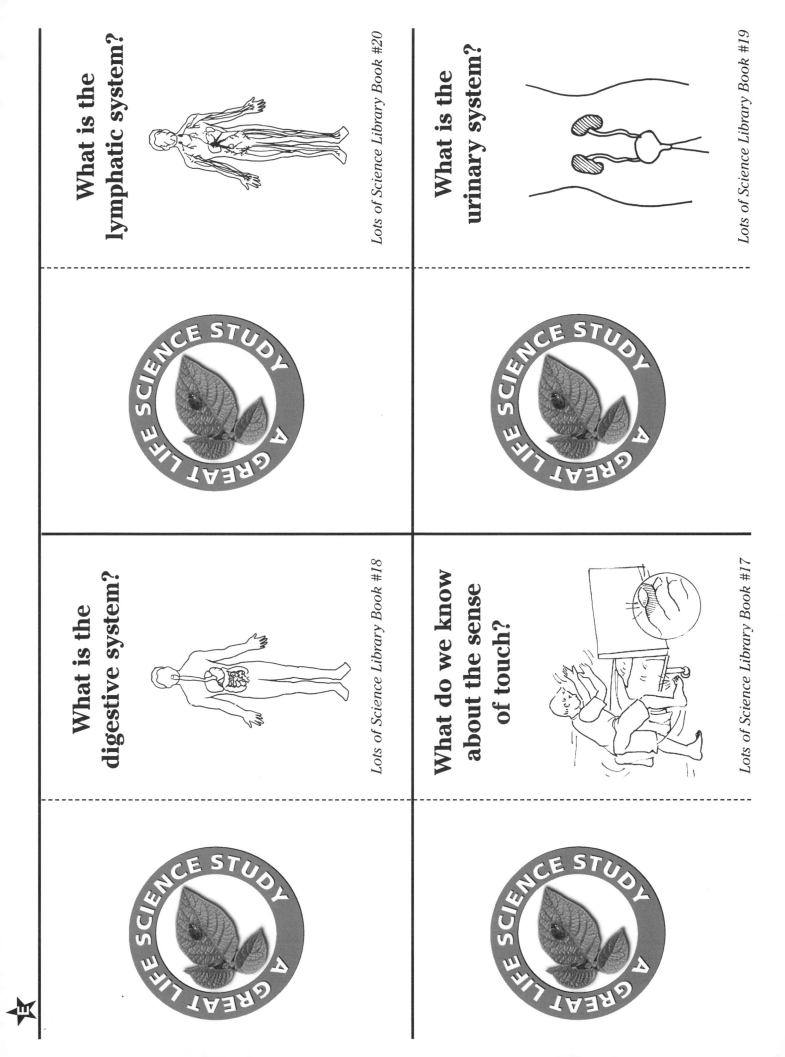

Lots of Science Library Book #20

What is the urinary system?

Lots of Science Library Book #19

What is the digestive system?

Lots of Science Library Book #18

What do we know about the sense of touch?

Lots of Science Library Book #17

drains
defends
carries
attack

* lymph
* lymph node
* lymph duct
* lymphocytes

Explain how the lymphatic system works in the human body.

digestion
hunger
teeth
saliva
stomach

* small intestines
* large intestines
* esophagus
* enzymes
* pancreas
* gall bladder
* villi

Explain how the digestion system works in the human body.

filters
cleaned
returned

* kidney
* ureter
* bladder
* urethra
* bile
* liver

Explain how the urinary system works in the human body.

touch
pain
danger
heat
blind

* temperature
* pressure

Explain the sense of touch in humans.

What do we know about new life?

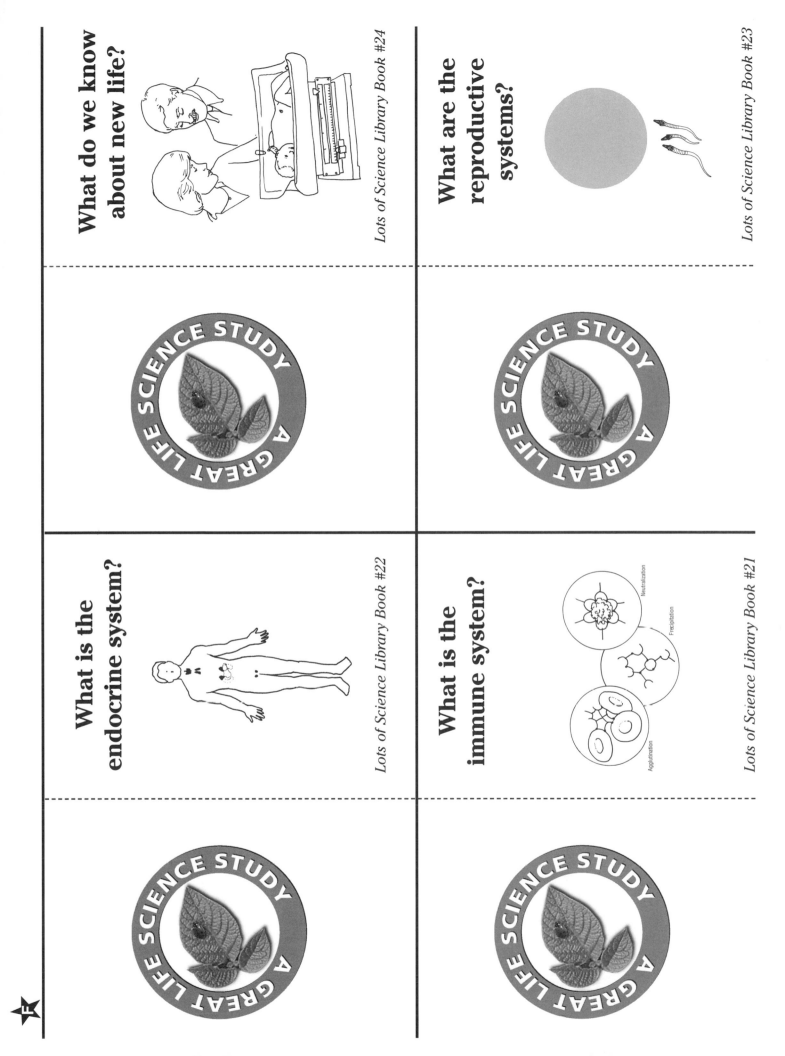

Lots of Science Library Book #24

What are the reproductive systems?

Lots of Science Library Book #23

What is the endocrine system?

Lots of Science Library Book #22

What is the immune system?

Neutralization

Precipitation

Agglutination

Lots of Science Library Book #21

F

---

join
cell
division
twins
DNA
* chromosomes
* genes
* placenta
* umbilical cord
* amniotic sac
* amniotic fluid

Explain how babies are
formed and grow through
gestation.

Describe how twins
are formed.

---

reproductive
baby
born
male
female
* ovaries
* fallopian tube
* uterus
* fertilization

Describe the male
reproductive system and
the female reproductive
system.

---

endocrine
messengers
* hypothalamus
* endocrine glands
* hormones
* pituitary glands

Explain how the endocrine
system works in the
human body.

---

immune
germs
disease
* phagocytes
* antibodies
* antigen
* vaccine

Explain how the immune
system works in the
human body.

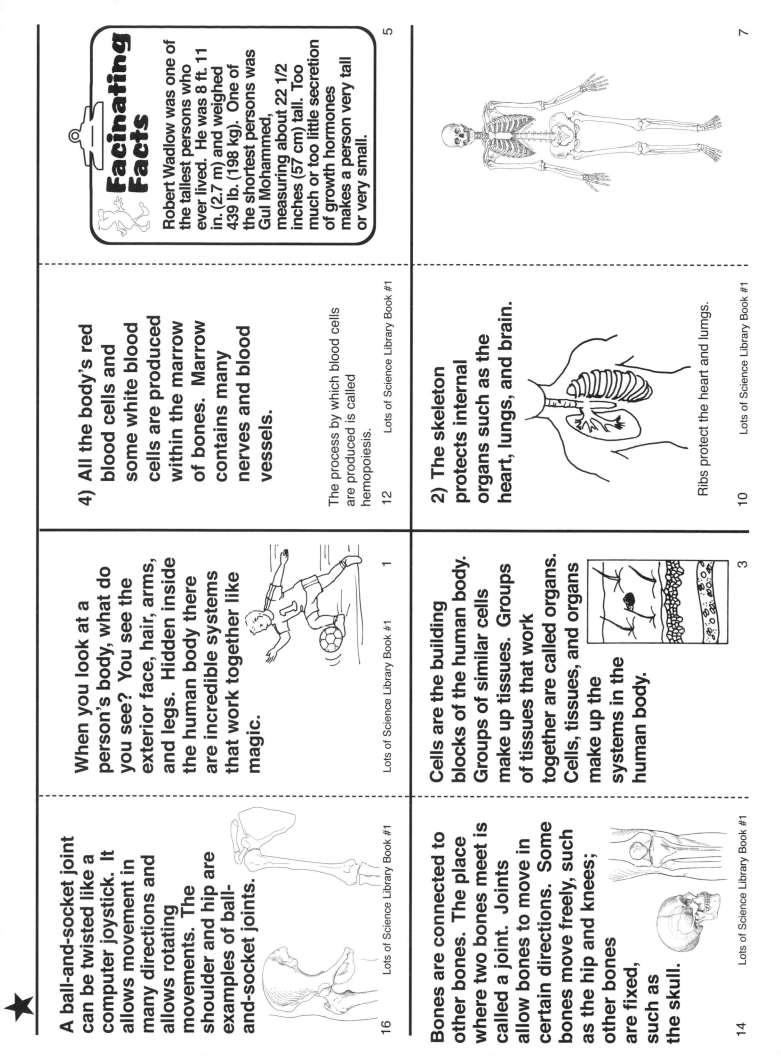

Facinating Facts

Robert Wadlow was one of the tallest persons who ever lived. He was 8 ft. 11 in. (2.7 m) and weighed 439 lb. (198 kg). One of the shortest persons was Gul Mohammed, measuring about 22 1/2 inches (57 cm) tall. Too much or too little secretion of growth hormones makes a person very tall or very small.

---

4) All the body's red blood cells and some white blood cells are produced within the marrow of bones. Marrow contains many nerves and blood vessels.

The process by which blood cells are produced is called hemopoiesis.

---

2) The skeleton protects internal organs such as the heart, lungs, and brain.

Ribs protect the heart and lumgs.

When you look at a person's body, what do you see? You see the exterior face, hair, arms, and legs. Hidden inside the human body there are incredible systems that work together like magic.

Cells are the building blocks of the human body. Groups of similar cells make up tissues. Groups of tissues that work together are called organs. Cells, tissues, and organs make up the systems in the human body.

A ball-and-socket joint can be twisted like a computer joystick. It allows movement in many directions and allows rotating movements. The shoulder and hip are examples of ball-and-socket joints.

Bones are connected to other bones. The place where two bones meet is called a joint. Joints allow bones to move in certain directions. Some bones move freely, such as the hip and knees; other bones are fixed, such as the skull.

This framework of bones is called a skeleton. All the bones and cartilage of the human body make up the skeletal system. Cartilage is similar to bone, but cartilage does not contain the mineral compounds found in bone. Therefore, cartilage is not as hard and brittle as bone. Cartilage is firm yet flexible. Your ears and the tip of your nose are made out of cartilage.

6

Lots of Science Library Book #1

The skeletal system provides four main functions:

1) The bones of the skeleton are arranged in such a manner to give the body shape and support.

9

Lots of Science Library Book #1

3) Bones anchor muscles to provide movement.

11

2

Lots of Science Library Book #1

The human body is supported by a framework of bones similar to the framework of a building. Like the beams of a building the size and shape of bones differ depending on their function and location. The human body is more amazing than the most spectacular building.

4

Lots of Science Library Book #1

There are two main types of moveable joints: hinge joint and ball-and-socket joint. The hinge joint moves in one direction only. A hinge joint is strong. The elbow and knee are examples of hinge joints.

elbow

knee

15

13

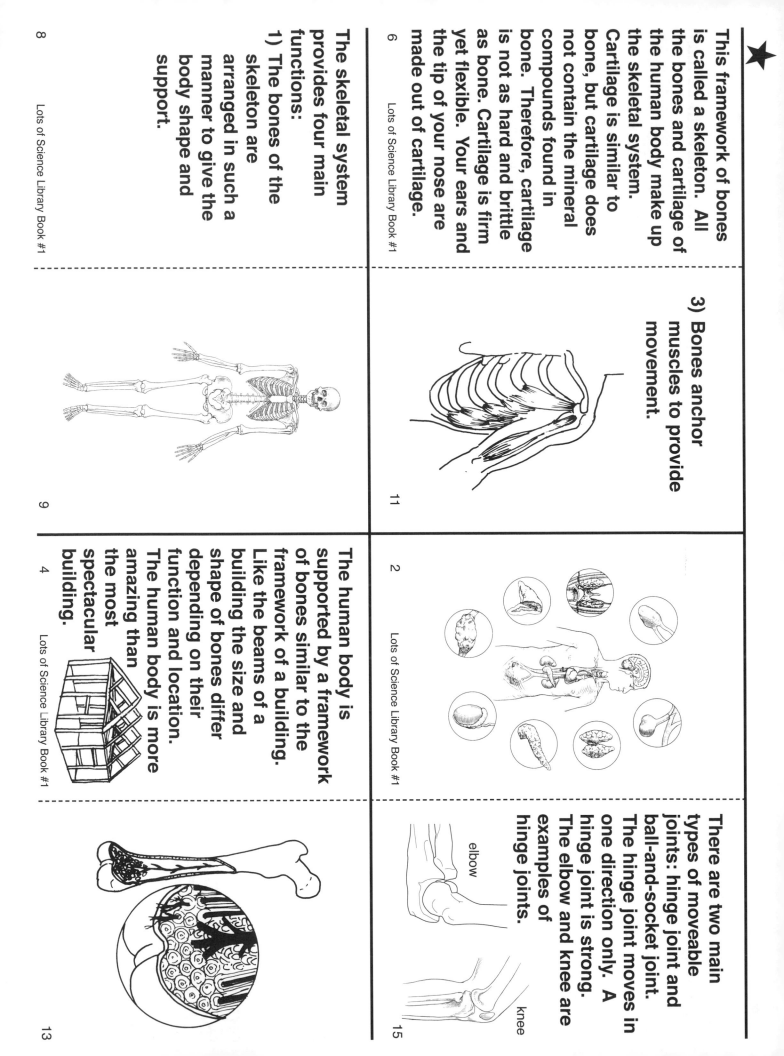

Bones have three main layers.
1) The outer layer is covered with a tough membrane which contains nerves and blood vessels. Special cells in the membrane help in the repair of bone injuries.

The outer membrane is called the periosteum. The cells which help repair bone injuries are called osteoblasts.

5

2) Beneath the tough membrane is a hard bony layer called compact bone. This consists of bone cells which release minerals that make bones hard. This layer is very strong and contains holes and channels carrying blood vessels and nerves to the inner layer of the bone.

7

However, if a person's diet lacks calcium, the bones release calcium into the blood to be carried to the other parts of the body that need it. If bones do not receive calcium to replenish their supply, bones become weak and brittle.

12   Lots of Science Library Book #2

Marrow contains many nerves and blood vessels. All the body's red blood cells are produced in the marrow. About 200 billion red blood cells are produced every day. Some white blood cells are also produced in the marrow.

The process by which blood cells are produced is called hemopoiesis. Some white blood cells finish maturing in other parts of the body.

10   Lots of Science Library Book #2

All the bones and cartilage in the human body make up the skeletal system. Bones develop from cartilage, the soft, rubbery material found in bones. The skeleton of a baby consists of 350 bones. These bones are still soft and fuse together as the baby grows.

1

Not all cartilage becomes bone. Some cartilage remains at the ends of bones for protection. The tip of your nose and your ears are made up of cartilage and will remain so throughout your life.

3

A doctor may treat a simple fracture on the arm or leg by wrapping it with a wet plaster bandage called a cast. The cast keeps the broken bones in place until the blood vessels and bone tissues grow together again. After it has healed, the bone is as strong as ever.

16   Lots of Science Library Book #2

Sometimes accidents may cause a bone to break. A broken bone is called a fracture. When this occurs, blood vessels also tear. Doctors usually take an X-ray to determine the location and type of fracture. Fractures may be simple, complete, or compound, among other types.

14   Lots of Science Library Book #2

The spongy bone is made up of tiny pieces of bone called trabeculae.

marrow.
hollow spaces in the sponge is filled with a soft jelly-like substance called bone marrow. The sponge is filled with a soft jelly-like substance called bone marrow.

3) At the end of bones is a spongy looking, but not soft, layer called spongy bone. Tiny pieces of bone form a design that looks like a honeycomb. The hollow spaces in the sponge is filled with a soft jelly-like substance called bone marrow.

Bones consists of calcium and phosphorus and smaller amounts of magnesium, and zinc.

Bones are made up of calcium and other minerals. Calcium, found in milk and dairy products, makes bones hard and strong. If a person's diet includes plenty of calcium, it is stored in the bones.

There are two types of bone marrow.
1) Red bone marrow produces red blood cells and is located at the ends of bones.

2) Yellow marrow consists mostly of fat and is located in the central hollow spaces of long bones.

Bone tissue is made up of living cells. Bones look hard and strong but are not as solid as they appear. They are designed to be strong, yet light in weight. Most bones are hollow in the middle, such as the bones in the arms and legs. About 50% of bone is water, and the remaining 50% consists of minerals and protein.

The process by which bone is formed is called osteogenesis or ossification.

As babies develop, minerals carried by blood vessels make the bones harder and stronger. Bone tissue begins developing at the center of the cartilage and gradually the bones grow. The skeleton of an adult human consists of 206 bones. About half of your bones are in your hands and feet.

Osteoporosis is a bone disease that affects many older people. The lack of calcium and vitamin D causes bones to become brittle.

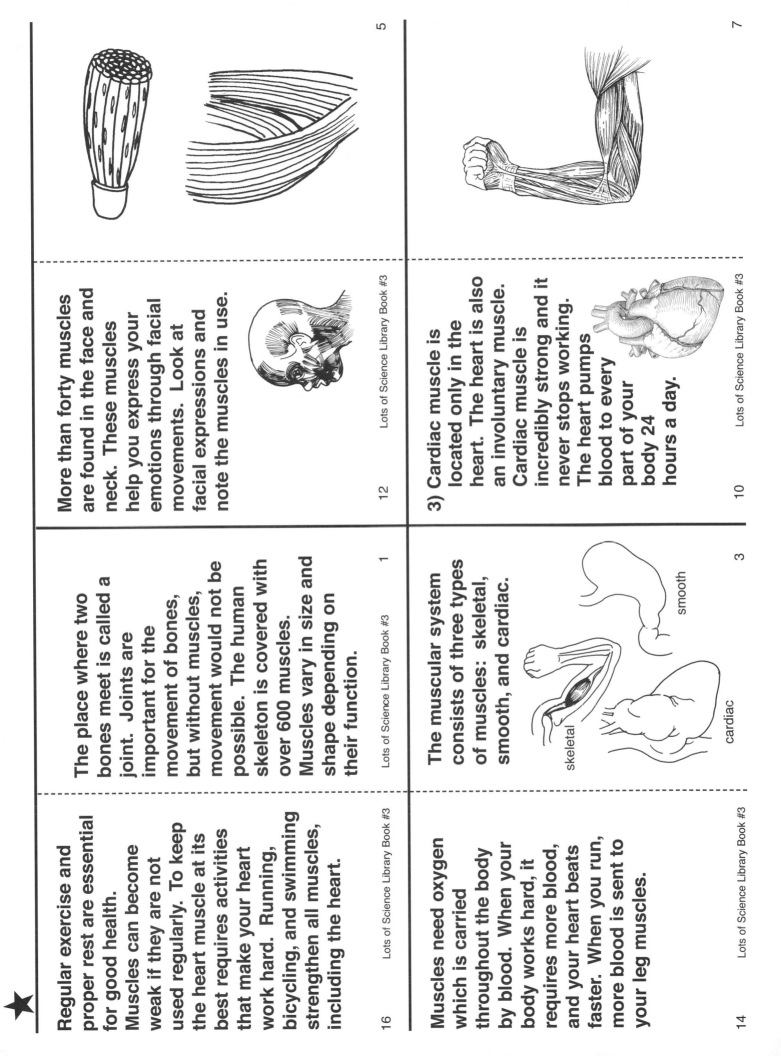

More than forty muscles are found in the face and neck. These muscles help you express your emotions through facial movements. Look at facial expressions and note the muscles in use.

---

3) Cardiac muscle is located only in the heart. The heart is also an involuntary muscle. Cardiac muscle is incredibly strong and it never stops working. The heart pumps blood to every part of your body 24 hours a day.

Regular exercise and proper rest are essential for good health. Muscles can become weak if they are not used regularly. To keep the heart muscle at its best requires activities that make your heart work hard. Running, bicycling, and swimming strengthen all muscles, including the heart.

The place where two bones meet is called a joint. Joints are important for the movement of bones, but without muscles, movement would not be possible. The human skeleton is covered with over 600 muscles. Muscles vary in size and shape depending on their function.

Muscles need oxygen which is carried throughout the body by blood. When your body works hard, it requires more blood, and your heart beats faster. When you run, more blood is sent to your leg muscles.

The muscular system consists of three types of muscles: skeletal, smooth, and cardiac.

skeletal

smooth

cardiac

Skeletal muscles are attached directly or indirectly to bones. Skeletal muscles work in pairs; one muscle contracts, and the other muscle relaxes. To raise your forearm, the bicep contracts and shortens as the tricep relaxes. To lower your forearm, the tricep contracts as the bicep relaxes.

Bones are held together at the joints by ligaments and cartilage. Ligaments are tough strands of elastic tissue located in joints to allow movement. A muscle is connected to a bone by tough elastic tissue called tendons. When the muscle contracts, the tendon pulls the bone resulting in movement.

Facinating Facts

The largest muscle in the human body is the gluteus maximus, which is the muscle you sit on. The smallest muscle is the stapedius located in the ear. Some of the strongest muscles are found in the jaw, and are used for biting.

---

2) Smooth muscles are located in the walls of internal organs and arteries. These muscles are used to force food through the intestines, pump blood through the arteries, and control the size of the iris in the eye. Smooth muscles are also called involuntary muscles because for the most part, you do not control them.

---

1) Skeletal muscles are also called voluntary muscles because you control these muscles. They are used to perform everyday movements such as lifting your arm or nodding your head. Skeletal muscles are made up of long, thin strands called muscle fibers. The fibers are bundled together by tissue containing blood vessels and nerves.

The bundles of muscles are called fascicles.

Bones and muscles are important and require good nutrition and exercise to maintain. To build muscle eat sensibly and make sure your diet includes foods rich in protein, such as meat, fish, legumes, eggs, and nuts. Include foods rich in calcium and vitamin D, such as dairy products and fish to strengthen bones.

Melanin is also produced mostly in the epidermis. Melanin is a pigment that determines skin color and absorbs damaging ultraviolet light. Some people have little melanin and are fair skinned. Other people have large amounts of melanin and have darker skin.

Albinism is a condition that occurs when no melanin is produced.

When skin is exposed to the sun, the body produces more melanin. This causes skin to darken. Sunlight is healthy for the skin because it produces vitamin D. However, too much sun may cause burns that lead to skin cancer. When in the sun, always wear sunscreen.

3) In the skin is a network of nerves that are sensitive to touch, pain, and temperature. Special organs throughout the body process light touch, heavy pressure, pain, heat, and cold. Some parts of the body have more sensory nerves than other parts.

Beneath the dermis is subcutaneous tissue, which contains fat and blood vessels. Hair follicles are located in the dermis and subcutaneous tissue.

Skin, hair, and nails make up the integumentary system. The skin is the human body's largest organ. Skin has three layers: epidermis, dermis, and subcutaneous tissue.

Oil produced in the skin keeps it waterproof and protects the body from germs. The human body is made up of 80% water and skin prevents rapid water loss.

After sweat evaporates, skin feels sticky because wastes remain on the skin including excess salt which sweat glands remove from the blood. It is important to bathe to remove these wastes.

Sweat glands are called sudoriferous glands.

4) Skin helps the body maintain its proper body temperature of 98.6 degrees F (37 degree C). As sweat evaporates, the body releases heat energy. Sweat usually occurs on the forehead and scalp first and then other parts of the body. Palms and soles are usually last.

dermis is the dermis, which is thicker than the epidermis. The dermis is strong and stretchy. It contains nerves that allow you to sense pressure, pain, and temperature. The dermis also protects internal organs.

Oil glands are called sebaceous

melanin

melanin

Skin has many functions:
1) Skin protects the body from injury and it protects the internal organs and other structures inside the human body. Skin is also waterproof and protects the body from drying out.
2) Skin is the human body's first line of defense against germs.

The epidermis is the outer layer of skin that you can see. It is made up of dead skin cells which are constantly being shed from the skin's surface and replaced by new cells.

The dermis contains blood vessels, elastic fibers, sweat glands, and oil glands. Oil glands produce oil that prevents the skin from drying out and help keep it waterproof. Oil glands are found everywhere on the body except the palms of the hands and soles of the feet.

Most of the cells in the epidermis produce keratin. Keratin is a tough, fibrous protein that helps to protect the skin from heat, germs, and chemicals. It also helps to keep the skin waterproof.

heat receptor
pressure receptors
touch receptors
cold receptor
hair root pressure receptor
pressure receptor

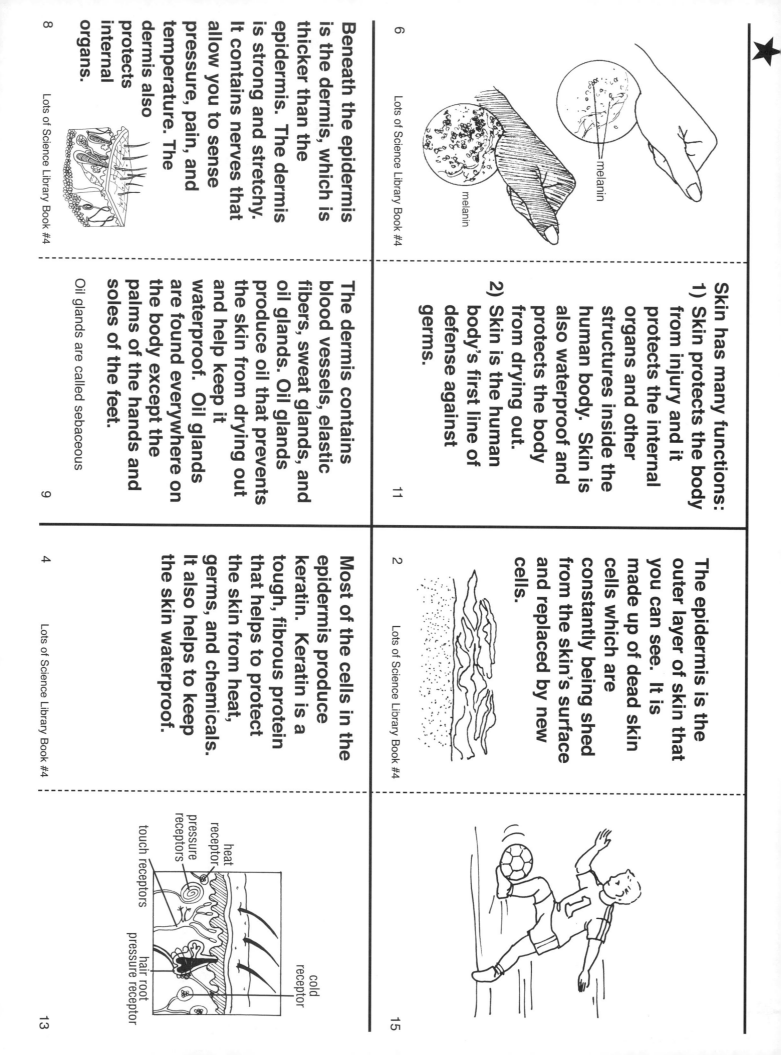

hair seen through microscope

Facinating Facts

When you are cold, goose bumps form on your skin. This occurs because the blood vessels squeeze deeper into your skin to prevent heat loss. Tiny muscles next to the hair follicles contract. The contraction pulls the follicle upright and makes the hair stand up.

The average head has about 100,000 hairs. Each hair grows about 1/100 inch daily. That means, altogether, the hairs on your head grow about 1,000 inches per day.

Each hair grows from a follicle. The shape of the follicle determines whether hair is straight or curly. A round follicle grows straight hair; an oval follicle grows wavy hair; and a flat follicle grows curly hair.

straight   wavy   curly

The integumentary system consists of skin, hair, and nails. An average adult has about four million hairs. The most obvious place to see hair is on your head. However, if you look closely, you will discover that your body is covered with fine hair except for your lips, palms, and soles.

Every hair on your body is connected to a nerve. These nerves touch receptors at hair roots and detect pressure, such as a pesky insect on your arm.

hair root
pressure receptor

Facinating Facts

The longest nail on record goes to Shridhar Chillal of India. His thumbnail measured 4 ft. 8 in. (1.4 m).

Nails are embedded in sensitive tissue to help the sense of touch. Nails grow at an average rate of about .02 inch (.5 mm) a week.

Every 3-5 years a hair root rests causing the hair to fall out, and new hair begins to grow. When you get a haircut, it does not hurt because only the root of the hair is living.

The base of a strand of hair is called a hair follicle. Cells in the follicle contain melanin, the same substance in skin. Melanin gives hair its color. As we age, hair may begin to look gray or white because pigment production slows down.

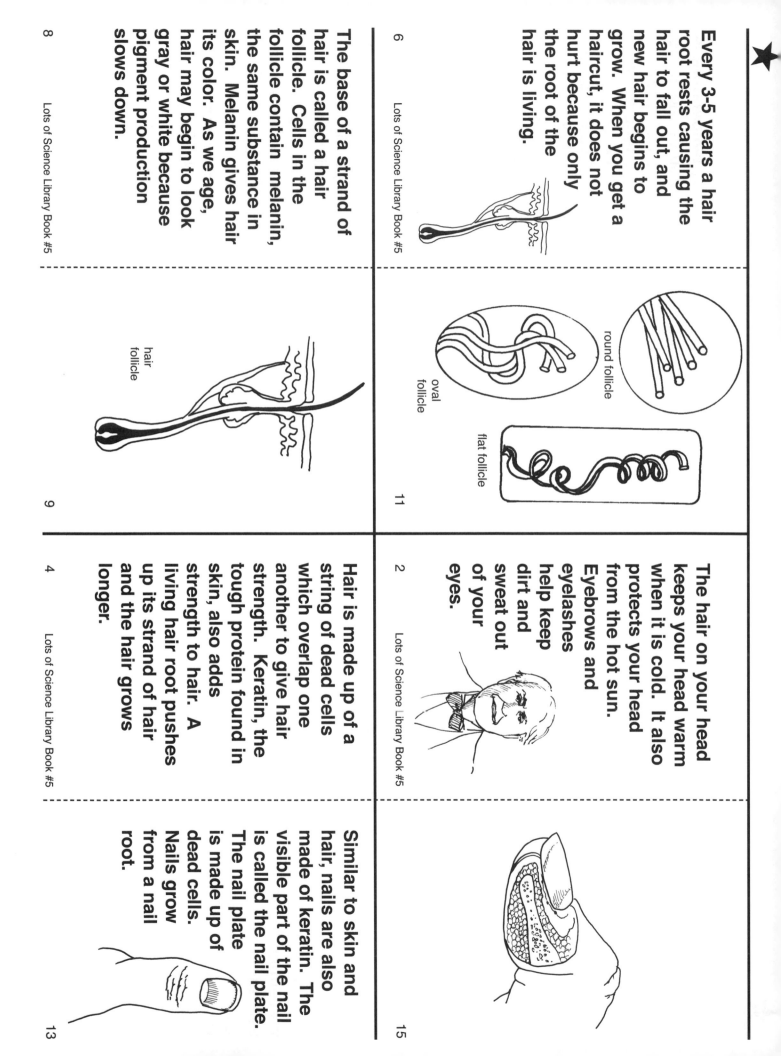

round follicle

oval follicle

flat follicle

---

hair follicle

The hair on your head keeps your head warm when it is cold. It also protects your head from the hot sun. Eyebrows and eyelashes help keep dirt and sweat out of your eyes.

Hair is made up of a string of dead cells which overlap one another to give hair strength. Keratin, the tough protein found in skin, also adds strength to hair. A living hair root pushes up its strand of hair and the hair grows longer.

Similar to skin and hair, nails are also made of keratin. The visible part of the nail is called the nail plate. The nail plate is made up of dead cells. Nails grow from a nail root.

2) Body temperature is regulated by the blood. Blood carries body heat throughout the body to keep it at a constant 98.6 degrees Fahrenheit (37 degrees Celsius). Blood carries heat from the internal organs to the skin.

When you are cold, your body needs to hold heat in, so blood flow is directed away from the skin. This is why you sometimes look pale when you feel cold.

White blood cells are colorless. Blood contains far fewer white blood cells than red blood cells, but white blood cells are very important. Their job is to protect the body from harmful agents, such as viruses, bacteria, and fungi, that can enter the body through the mouth or cuts in the skin.

Three main types of white blood cells are neutrophils, monocytes, and lymphocytes.

Red blood cells give blood its red color. The main function of red blood cells is to carry oxygen from the lungs to the body's cells. Blood travels from the lungs to the body's tissues and back to the lungs again in about a minute.

Every red blood cell consists of hemoglobin, which gives blood its red color. Hemoglobin is a special protein that picks up oxygen and releases it where it is needed.

The cardiovascular system consists of the heart, blood vessels, and blood. Blood is the only liquid tissue.

Blood plasma helps to maintain proper blood pressure and is important in the exchange of fluids. Most substances carried by blood are carried in the plasma. This includes nutrients, waste, and hormones.

When you exhale, carbon dioxide is released as a waste product and carried by red blood cells and plasma to the lungs, where it is exhaled.

---

1 cut in the skin
2 platelets collect
3 clot forms
4 scab is formed

Platelets, which are fragments of cells, help blood clot preventing excessive loss of blood. When an injury occurs, platelets quickly collect to form a "plug."

Platelets do not have a nucleus. They live for about 8-14 days.

3) When the body receives an injury or cut that damages blood vessels, blood can thicken to form a lump, called a clot, to help stop the bleeding. Blood also contains special proteins called antibodies to help protect the body against disease.

When you feel hot, the blood vessels in your skin expand, allowing more blood to flow near the surface of the skin where heat is lost. This is why your face sometimes looks red when you feel hot.

Red blood cells last for about 120 days. Their many trips through the body cause them to break down so they can't carry oxygen. Two million red blood cells are produced every second. Both red and white blood cells are produced in bone marrow.

The three main parts of blood are red blood cells, white blood cells, and platelets. One drop of blood contains about 5 million red blood cells; 8,000 white blood cells; and 250,000 platelets.

An average adult's body contains about 10.6 pints (5 L) of blood. Blood is about 55% plasma and 45% blood cells. Plasma is the liquid part of blood. Plasma is about 95% water and 5% proteins, salts, and other substances.

Blood has three main functions: transportation, regulation, and protection. **1)** Blood carries oxygen from the lungs to all the cells of the body. It also carries carbon dioxide from these cells to the lungs to be eliminated. Blood carries nutrients from the stomach and intestines to cells and it carries waste products away from cells.

A clot of thick blood forms, and white blood cells begin to destroy harmful bacteria. When the clot dries, a scab is formed, allowing time for the tissue to repair itself.

Most white blood cells last for a few weeks. White blood cells last for only a few hours if they are fighting an invasion. Another type of white blood cell that releases antibodies that target bacteria and viruses can last for years.

The latter cells are called lymphocytes.

The human body needs oxygen to live. It also needs to get rid of carbon dioxide. When you breathe in, or inhale, your lungs take in oxygen and when you breathe out, or exhale, your lungs give off carbon dioxide.

5

---

① blood enters the right atrium

② valve opens, the deoxygenated blood moves to the right ventricle

③ deoxygenated blood pumps through the pulmonary arteries to the lungs where it is cleansed of carbon dioxide and filled with oxygen

7

Veins carry oxygen-depleted blood back to the heart. The walls of veins are thin and contain valves to prevent the blood from flowing backward due to gravity and low pressure.

vein

Note: The pulmonary veins carry oxygenated blood back to the heart.

12

There are two types of blood vessels; arteries and veins. Both arteries and veins branch out in the body becoming smaller and smaller vessels.

vein

artery

10

The human body contains a network of tubes called blood vessels.

circulatory system

1

The heart is the center of the cardiovascular system. It is located in the middle of the chest between the two lungs. The heart is about the size of a fist.

3

Facinating Facts

During an average person's life span, the heart pumps blood throughout the body over 2 billion times.

16

As the heart beats, blood surges through the arteries. This surge, called a pulse, can be detected at certain points on your body.

temples
neck
crook of elbow
wrist
groin
inside back of ankle
back of knee
top of foot

14

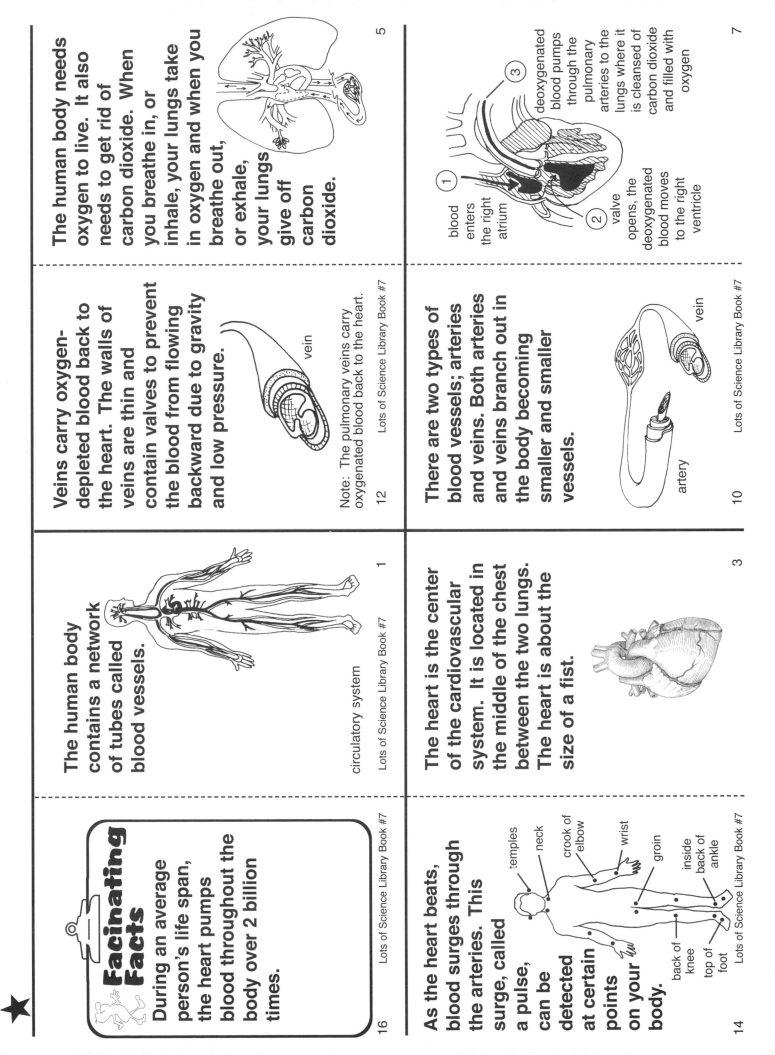

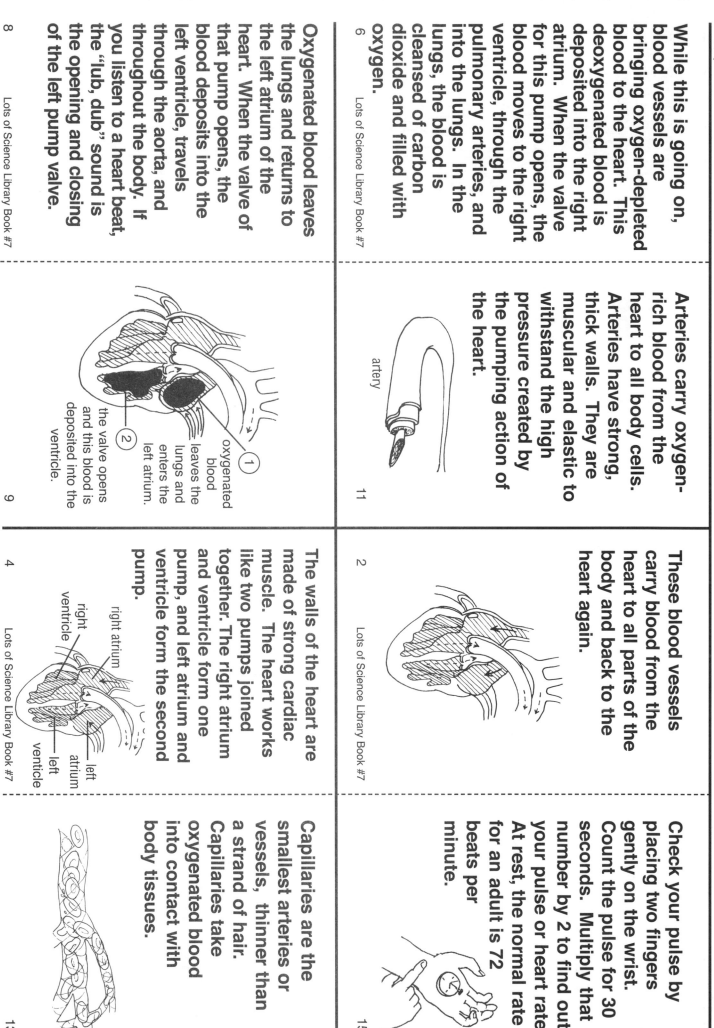

While this is going on, blood vessels are bringing oxygen-depleted blood to the heart. This deoxygenated blood is deposited into the right atrium. When the valve for this pump opens, the blood moves to the right ventricle, through the pulmonary arteries, and into the lungs. In the lungs, the blood is cleansed of carbon dioxide and filled with oxygen.

Oxygenated blood leaves the lungs and returns to the heart. When the valve of that pump opens, the blood deposits into the left ventricle, travels through the aorta, and throughout the body. If you listen to a heart beat, the "lub, dub" sound is the opening and closing of the left pump valve.

Arteries carry oxygen-rich blood from the heart to all body cells. Arteries have strong, thick walls. They are muscular and elastic to withstand the high pressure created by the pumping action of the heart.

artery

oxygenated blood leaves the lungs and enters the left atrium.

the valve opens and this blood is deposited into the ventricle.

These blood vessels carry blood from the heart to all parts of the body and back to the heart again.

The walls of the heart are made of strong cardiac muscle. The heart works like two pumps joined together. The right atrium and ventricle form one pump, and left atrium and ventricle form the second pump.

right atrium

right ventricle

left atrium

left ventricle

Check your pulse by placing two fingers gently on the wrist. Count the pulse for 30 seconds. Multiply that number by 2 to find out your pulse or heart rate. At rest, the normal rate for an adult is 72 beats per minute.

Capillaries are the smallest arteries or vessels, thinner than a strand of hair. Capillaries take oxygenated blood into contact with body tissues.

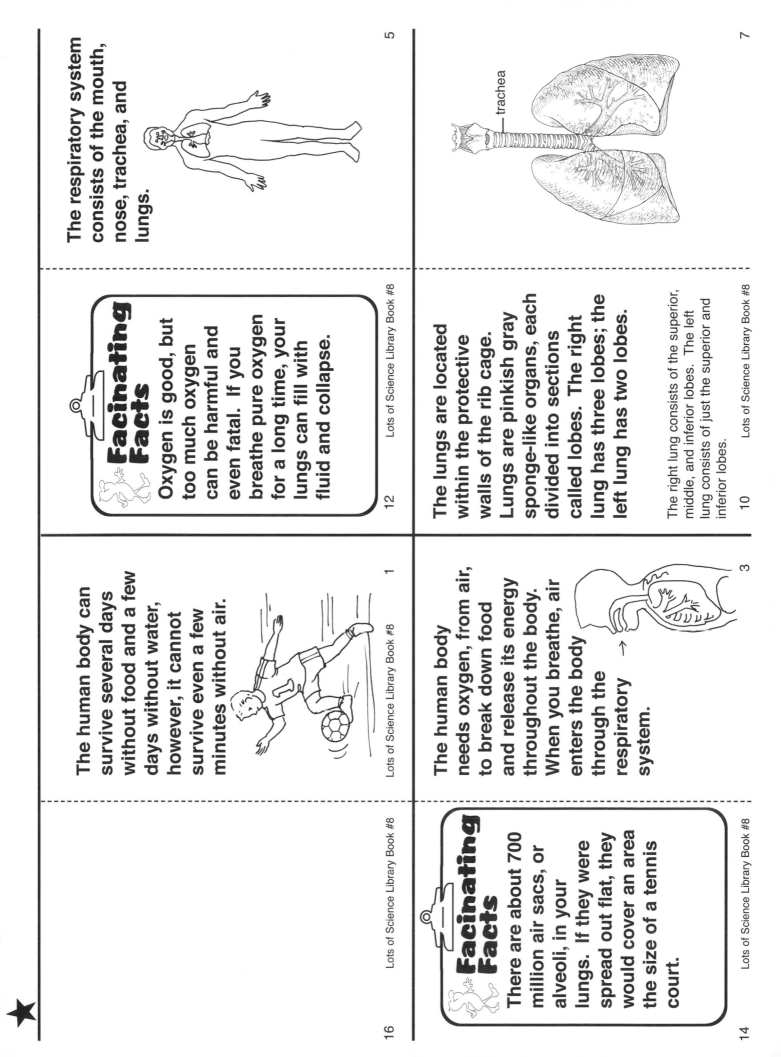

The respiratory system consists of the mouth, nose, trachea, and lungs.

5

trachea

7

Oxygen is good, but too much oxygen can be harmful and even fatal. If you breathe pure oxygen for a long time, your lungs can fill with fluid and collapse.

12   Lots of Science Library Book #8

The lungs are located within the protective walls of the rib cage. Lungs are pinkish gray sponge-like organs, each divided into sections called lobes. The right lung has three lobes; the left lung has two lobes.

The right lung consists of the superior, middle, and inferior lobes. The left lung consists of just the superior and inferior lobes.

10   Lots of Science Library Book #8

The human body can survive several days without food and a few days without water, however, it cannot survive even a few minutes without air.

1

Lots of Science Library Book #8

16

The human body needs oxygen, from air, to break down food and release its energy throughout the body. When you breathe, air enters the body through the respiratory system.

3

There are about 700 million air sacs, or alveoli, in your lungs. If they were spread out flat, they would cover an area the size of a tennis court.

Lots of Science Library Book #8

14

The main organs of the respiratory system are the lungs. The windpipe, or trachea, divides into two main airways which lead to the right and left lungs.

The two main airways are called bronchi.

The clusters of air sacs are called

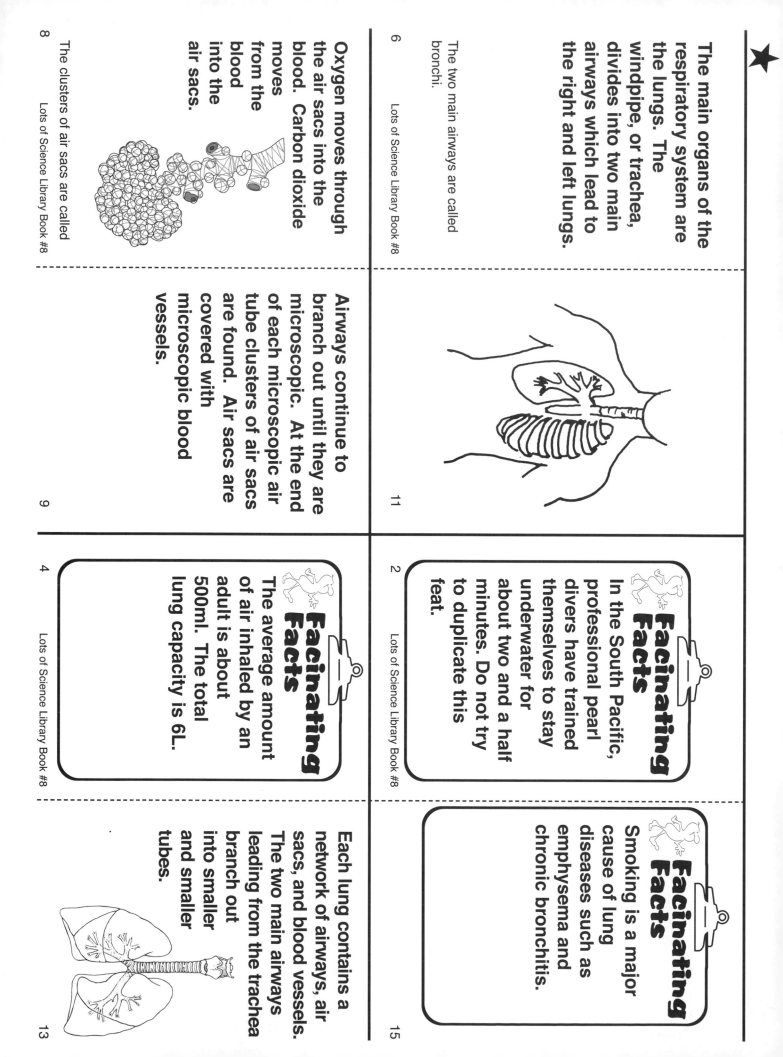

Oxygen moves through the air sacs into the blood. Carbon dioxide moves from the blood into the air sacs.

Airways continue to branch out until they are microscopic. At the end of each microscopic air tube clusters of air sacs are found. Air sacs are covered with microscopic blood vessels.

Facinating Facts

In the South Pacific, professional pearl divers have trained themselves to stay underwater for about two and a half minutes. Do not try to duplicate this feat.

Facinating Facts

The average amount of air inhaled by an adult is about 500ml. The total lung capacity is 6L.

Facinating Facts

Smoking is a major cause of lung diseases such as emphysema and chronic bronchitis.

Each lung contains a network of airways, air sacs, and blood vessels. The two main airways leading from the trachea branch out into smaller and smaller tubes.

Facinating Facts

During the late 19th and early 20th centuries when corsets were fashionable, it was not uncommon for women to faint due to lack of oxygen. Corsets squeezed their lungs and diaphragm making it impossible to breathe properly.

Facinating Facts

Hiccups occur when the stomach presses on the diaphragm. This irritates the diaphragm and causes involuntary contractions. This action causes the vocal cords to close rapidly and produces the 'hic' in hiccups.

The muscle under your lungs is called the diaphragm. When you inhale, the diaphragm moves down and the ribs move out.

The food you eat and the air you breathe create energy your body needs to stay alive. This process produces a build-up of carbon dioxide that is poisonous, so your body needs to get rid of it.

When you inhale, you breathe in oxygen. When you exhale, you release carbon dioxide.

Facinating Facts

Yawning occurs when the body has rising carbon dioxide levels. By yawning, the body takes in a large amount of oxygen, to replace carbon dioxide in the lungs.

When your body is at rest, you do not require as much energy and oxygen as when you are active. When an adult is resting, he breathes about 12-18 times a minute.

The process of cleansing carbon dioxide from the blood and adding oxygen to the blood, is called gas exchange.

Oxygen from the air you inhale goes into your lungs, through your heart, and is carried to many cells where it is used to create energy.

When you exhale, the diaphragm moves up, and the ribs move back. This movement causes the air in the lungs to squeeze out.

The cardiovascular and respiratory systems work together. Arteries carry oxygenated blood away from the heart and veins carry blood containing carbon dioxide to the lungs where it is exhaled.

When you inhale, or breathe in, air enters your mouth or nose and goes down the trachea. The end of the trachea splits into two airways that carry air to the right and left lungs. The airways are called bronchi. (Singular is bronchus.)

Your body requires more oxygen when you run, so your breathing rate is increased.

Fascinating Facts

Singers and trumpet players learn to use their diaphragm for good air control.

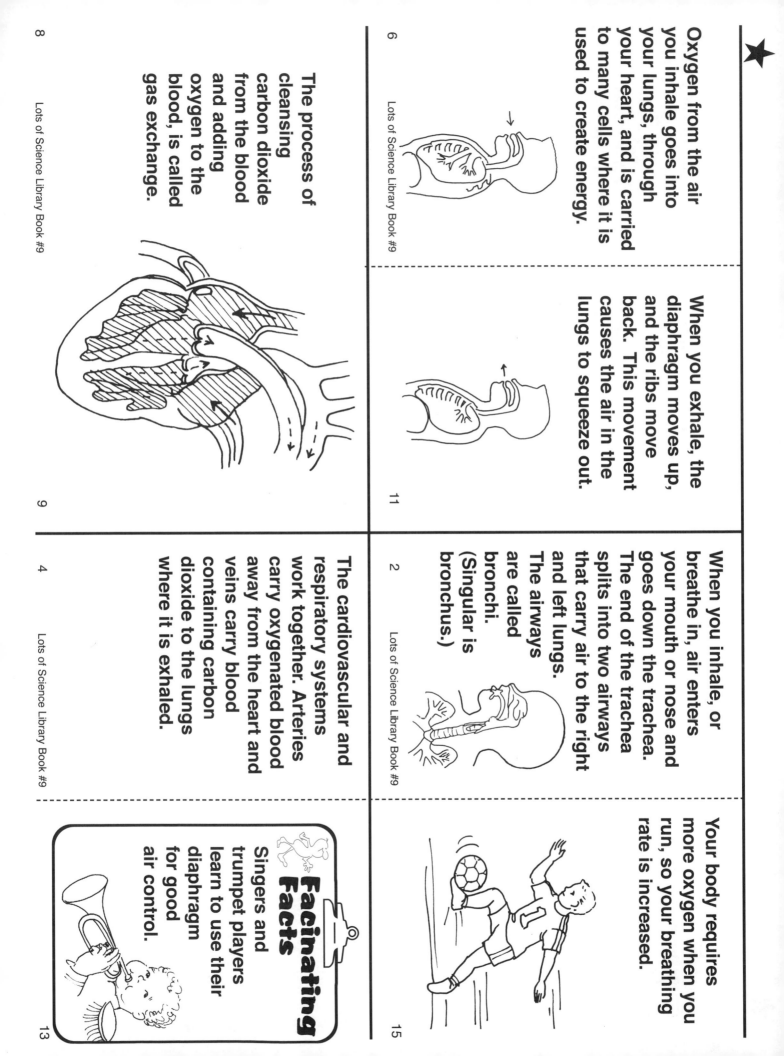

When you touch a hot object, you quickly pull away. This is called a reflex, or automatic response. Reflexes keep you safe by making quick movements in physically threatening situations.

5

The nervous system is divided into two parts:
1) The central nervous system (CNS), is the brain and spinal cord.

7

Axons send information from the neuron. Every neuron has only one axon. Axons are thin and long.

dendrites
cell body
axon

12

The cell body of each neuron contains the nucleus, and strands called nerve fibers.

dendrites
cell body
axon

10

Everyday activities such as walking, breathing, dreaming, feeling pain, or solving problems involve the nervous system.

1

Although the brain is often compared to a computer, the human brain is far more complex than any computer. Weighing only about 3 lb. (1.4 kg), it is the major organ of the nervous system.

3

The involuntary nervous system helps the body perform its automatic functions, such as breathing, heart beating, and digesting food. That is why you don't have to think about breathing; your body does it for you automatically.

16

The peripheral nervous system (PNS) is divided into two systems:

1) voluntary

2) involuntary

The voluntary system is called the somatic nervous system; the involuntary is called the autonomic nervous system

14

8

Reflexes occur when pain sensors send messages to and from the spinal cord. The brain is not directly involved; it receives the messages after the reflex takes place.

---

2) The peripheral nervous system (PNS) consists of the nerves connecting the brain and spinal cord to other parts of the body. The PNS sends messages between the CNS and the rest of the body.

6

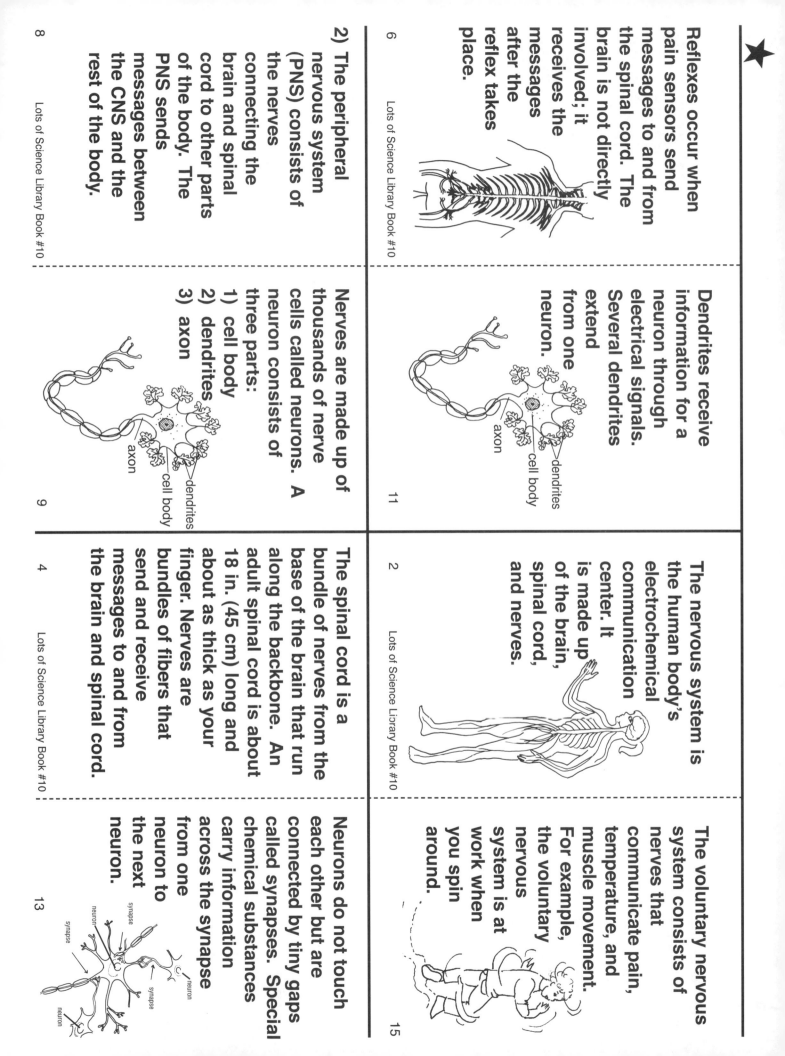

Dendrites receive information for a neuron through electrical signals. Several dendrites extend from one neuron.

(diagram labels: axon, cell body, dendrites)

11

Nerves are made up of thousands of nerve cells called neurons. A neuron consists of three parts:

1) cell body
2) dendrites
3) axon

(diagram labels: axon, cell body, dendrites)

9

The nervous system is the human body's electrochemical communication center. It is made up of the brain, spinal cord, and nerves.

2

The spinal cord is a bundle of nerves from the base of the brain that run along the backbone. An adult spinal cord is about 18 in. (45 cm) long and about as thick as your finger. Nerves are bundles of fibers that send and receive messages to and from the brain and spinal cord.

4

Neurons do not touch each other but are connected by tiny gaps called synapses. Special chemical substances carry information across the synapse from one neuron to the next neuron.

(diagram labels: neuron, synapse, synapse, synapse, neuron, neuron)

13

The voluntary nervous system consists of nerves that communicate pain, temperature, and muscle movement. For example, the voluntary nervous system is at work when you spin around.

15

The cerebrum consists of two parts, the right and left cerebral hemispheres. The two hemispheres are joined by a bridge made up of a bundle of nerves. The cerebrum makes up about 85% of the brain's weight.

The bundle of nerves connecting the right and left hemispheres is called the corpus callosum.

folds and creases in the cortex

---

4) The occipital lobe is primarily involved in vision. The occipital lobe is located at the back of the head.

occipital

2) The temporal lobe is involved in hearing and memory. The temporal lobe is located above the ears.

temporal

The brain is the most important part of the human body's nervous system. It is also the control center for all body activities, including thinking, memory, emotions, dreaming, walking, talking, tasting… everything you do.

The brain consists of the cerebellum, cerebrum, and the brainstem. The brainstem merges into the top of the spinal cord.

cerebellum

cerebrum

brainstem

Most people are right-handed because the left hemisphere controls language. For left-handed people the right side of the brain controls language.

The right side of the brain is used to process perceptual concepts. If you had to pack your luggage in the trunk of your car, your right brain is used to visualize the best way to accomplish the task.

The outer layer of the cerebrum is the cortex. The cortex is where processes such as thinking, reasoning, learning, and memory take place. The cortex is about 1/6 in. (2-4 mm) thick. Due to the cortex's folds and creases, more nerve cells are packed together.

Each hemisphere of the cerebrum is divided into four parts called lobes.

1) frontal lobe

2) temporal lobe

3) parietal lobe

4) occipital lobe

3) The parietal lobe is involved in body awareness and interpreting senses. The parietal lobe is located at the top of the head toward the rear.

parietal

11

The brain uses large amounts of energy and needs a constant supply of blood. If brain cells do not receive blood for as little as five minutes, they die due to lack of oxygen.

2

The left side of the brain is used primarily for language and speech. Therefore, the left side of your brain reads the word 'dog,' and then the right side enables you to see a picture of a dog in your mind.

15

1) The frontal lobe is involved in the control of voluntary muscles, intelligence, and personality. The frontal lobe is located behind the forehead.

frontal

9

The cerebellum maintains balance and the coordination of body movements.

4

In the brainstem, the nerves from the left and right hemispheres change sides. Therefore, the left hemisphere controls the right side of the body; the right hemisphere controls the left side.

The right and left hemispheres of the brain are joined by the corpus callosum.

13

The human eye has often been compared to a camera but, like the entire human body, it is vastly more complex. When light strikes an object, light enters the eye and passes into the pupil.

light

5

The cornea is a clear thin disc in front of the eye. As light enters the eye, the curved surface of the cornea bends the light to focus the image at the back of the eye.

—cornea

7

An image on the retina appears upside-down. This is because the lens bends the light rays toward each other where they eventually cross. The image is then turned right-side up at the optic nerve.

We experience the world through our senses: sight, sound, taste, touch, and smell. To understand the sense of sight, we must first look at the properties of light which make vision possible.

The colored part of the eye is called the iris. People may have blue, green, or brown eyes, or a blend of colors. The pupil is the black center of the iris.

pupil
iris

3

Facinating Facts

Eye Expressions

"We see eye to eye."
We agree.

"I turned a blind eye."
I ignored something.

"Keep your eyes peeled."
Look out.

"...in the mind's eye..."
This refers to the imagination.

Gradually move the page toward you until the circle disappears. To find the blind spot in your right eye, repeat the process covering your left eye, and staring at the circle until the square disappears.

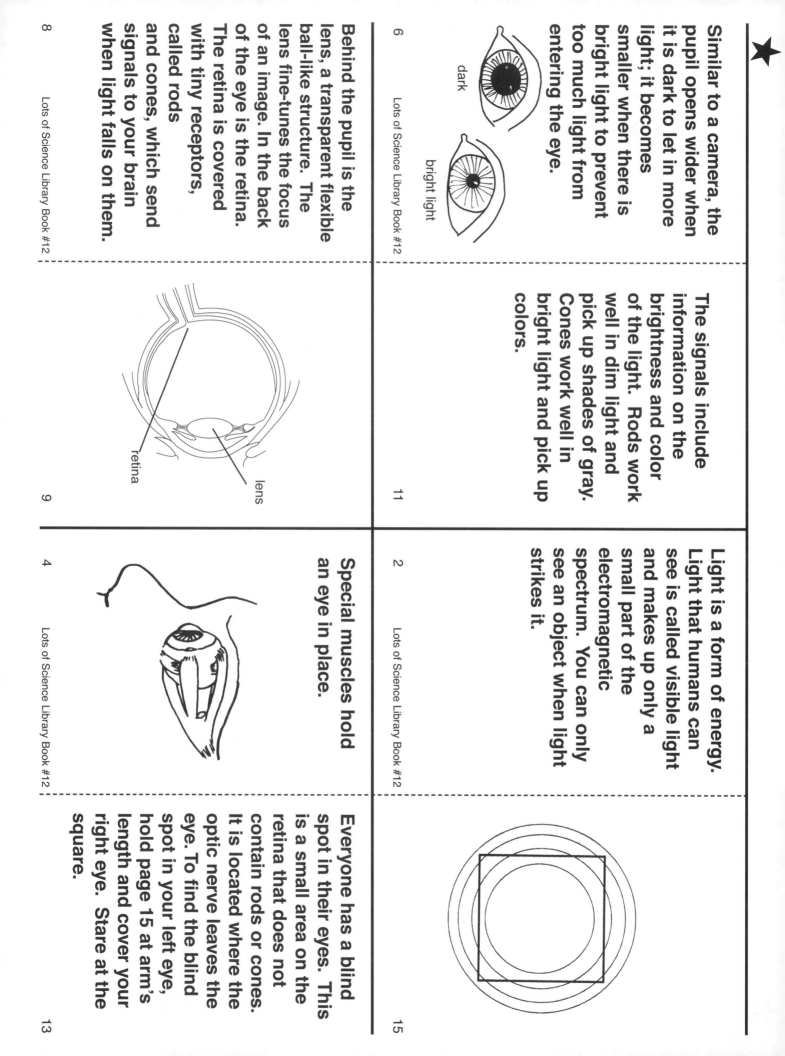

Similar to a camera, the pupil opens wider when it is dark to let in more light; it becomes smaller when there is bright light to prevent too much light from entering the eye.

6

dark

bright light

Lots of Science Library Book #12

8

Behind the pupil is the lens, a transparent flexible ball-like structure. The lens fine-tunes the focus of an image. In the back of the eye is the retina. The retina is covered with tiny receptors, called rods and cones, which send signals to your brain when light falls on them.

retina

lens

9

The signals include information on the brightness and color of the light. Rods work well in dim light and pick up shades of gray. Cones work well in bright light and pick up colors.

11

Light is a form of energy. Light that humans can see is called visible light and makes up only a small part of the electromagnetic spectrum. You can only see an object when light strikes it.

2

Lots of Science Library Book #12

Special muscles hold an eye in place.

4

Lots of Science Library Book #12

Everyone has a blind spot in their eyes. This is a small area on the retina that does not contain rods or cones. It is located where the optic nerve leaves the eye. To find the blind spot in your left eye, hold page 15 at arm's length and cover your right eye. Stare at the square.

15

13

Can you see a young blonde woman wearing a dark hat or an older man with a mustache?

Your brain also perceives shape and brightness constancies. Although a tomato looks different in bright light than in dim light, your brain recognizes the shape and color of a tomato.

When an object is far away from you, it appears smaller than when it is close to you. Your brain recognizes this fact and perceives close and distant objects, such as the trees on the next page, similar in size. This is called size contancy in the brain.

Sight is different than perception. Sight is what you see; perception is how your brain processes what is seen. For this reason, two people can see the same object and perceive different things. Look at the picture on the next page.

What do you perceive in the object? Ask someone else to look at the object and tell you what he/she perceives. Look at the object again. Your perception may shift from a single goblet to two silhouettes.

---

square 2

square 3

Two of the same objects can be perceived as different images because each is in a different context. This is called an optical illusion. Which of these lines is longer? Use your ruler to test your idea.

Line "A"

Line "B"

6

If you have difficulty seeing both images, focus on the area indicated by the arrow and try to see it as a nose the first time and as a chin the next time. By doing this, the images will shift from the old man to the young woman.

Lots of Science Library Book #13

8

Even a simple line picture can be perceived as one of two images. This happens because there are no features strong enough for your brain to conclude which one is correct. This picture can be either a duck or a rabbit.

Lots of Science Library Book #13

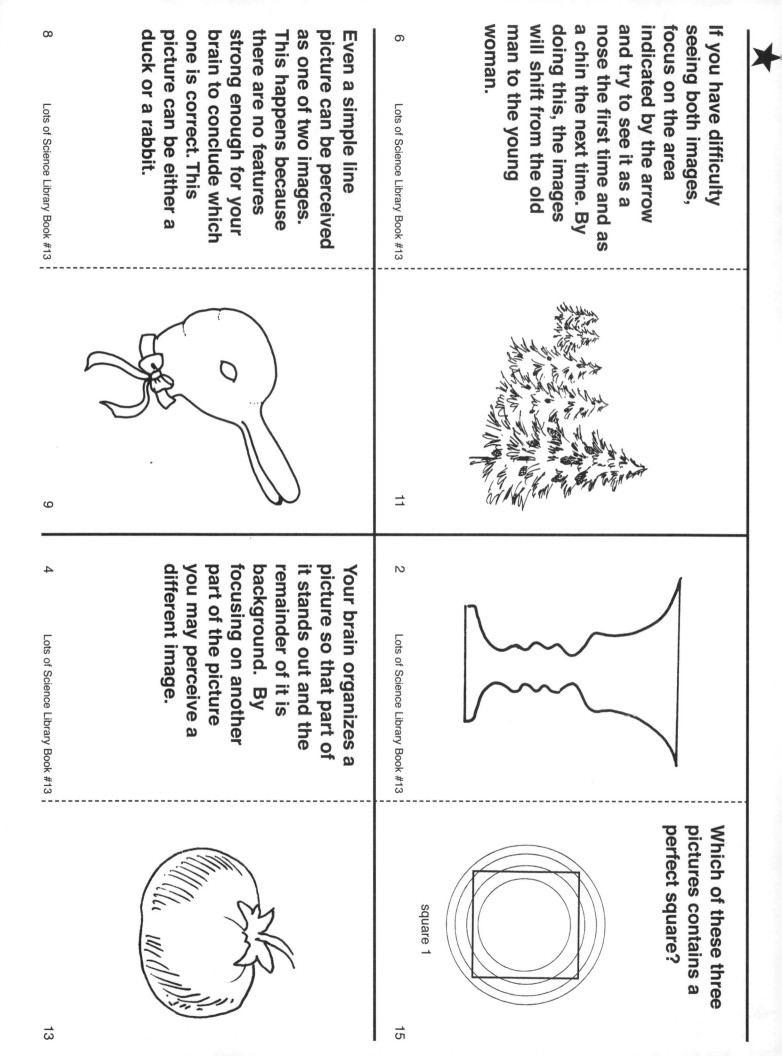

9

11

2

Your brain organizes a picture so that part of it stands out and the remainder of it is background. By focusing on another part of the picture you may perceive a different image.

Lots of Science Library Book #13

4

a different image.

Lots of Science Library Book #13

13

15

square 1

Which of these three pictures contains a perfect square?

The human ear is made up of three parts: outer ear, middle ear, and inner ear. The outer ear consists of the auricle, the part of the ear that you can see. The auricle is flexible because it is made up of cartilage, a flexible, elastic tissue.

Sound waves move to the middle ear, which consists of the eardrum and three tiny bones -- hammer, anvil, and stirrup. The eardrum is a thin membrane that vibrates when sound waves strike it.

The eardrum is called the tympanic membrane.

The inner ear also contains special organs for balance. Without these organs, even a simple activity like walking would be nearly impossible.

The organs for balance consists of the semicircular canals and the vestibule.

The inner ear contains a coiled tube called the cochlea. Inside the cochlea are delicate, microscopic hairs that help change sound waves into electrical signals. These electrical signals travel along the auditory nerve to the brain.

You experience and learn about the world around you not only by sight, but also by sound. The human ear is the body's sound collector.

Sounds can be high-pitched or low-pitched because of different frequencies.

low-pitched

high-pitched

Frequency is measured in Hertz (Hz).

People who are deaf often learn to read lips or use sign language.

means "I love you"

Facinating Facts

When you spin around you feel dizzy because the fluid in the ear continues spinning even after you have stopped spinning.

★

The shape of the auricle helps collect sound waves. Sound waves continue to travel through the ear canal.

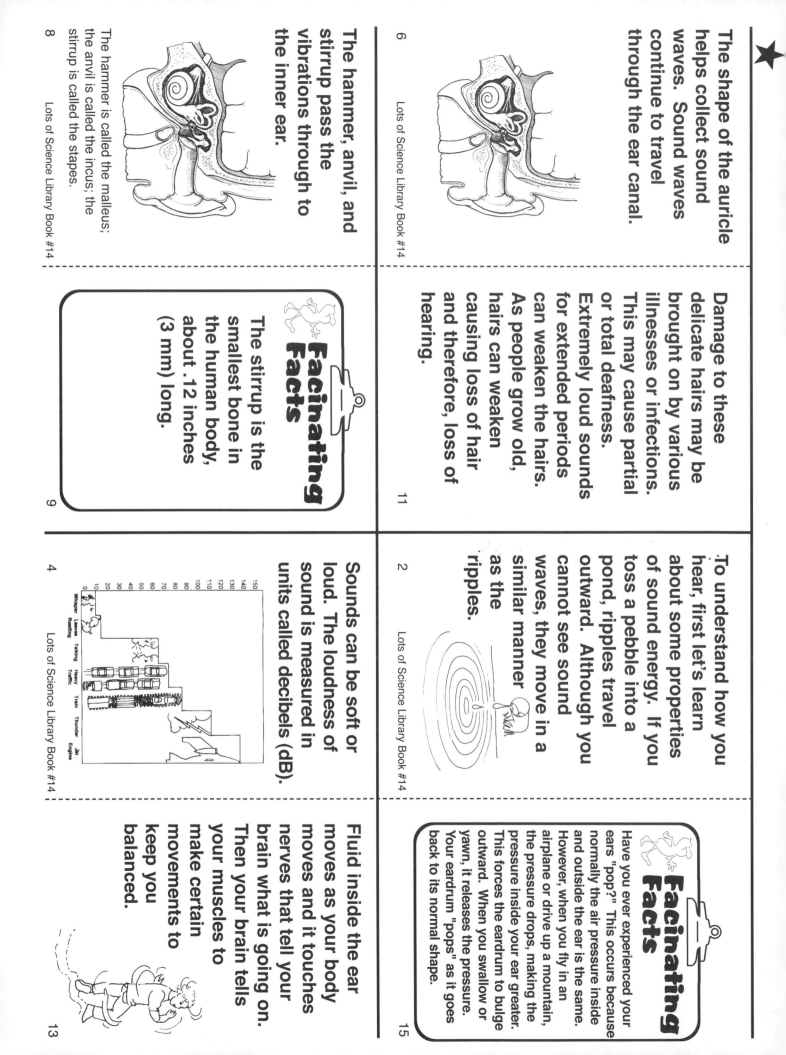

The hammer, anvil, and stirrup pass the vibrations through to the inner ear.

The hammer is called the malleus; the anvil is called the incus; the stirrup is called the stapes.

Damage to these delicate hairs may be brought on by various illnesses or infections. This may cause partial or total deafness. Extremely loud sounds for extended periods can weaken the hairs. As people grow old, hairs can weaken causing loss of hair and therefore, loss of hearing.

Facinating Facts

The stirrup is the smallest bone in the human body, about .12 inches (3 mm) long.

To understand how you hear, first let's learn about some properties of sound energy. If you toss a pebble into a pond, ripples travel outward. Although you cannot see sound waves, they move in a similar manner as the ripples.

Sounds can be soft or loud. The loudness of sound is measured in units called decibels (dB).

150
140
130
120
110
100
90
80
70
60
50
40
30
20
10
0

Whisper, Leaves Rustling, Talking, Heavy Traffic, Train, Thunder, Jet Engine

Fluid inside the ear moves as your body moves and it touches nerves that tell your brain what is going on. Then your brain tells your muscles to make certain movements to keep you balanced.

Facinating Facts

Have you ever experienced your ears "pop?" This occurs because normally the air pressure inside and outside the ear is the same. However, when you fly in an airplane or drive up a mountain, the pressure drops, making the pressure inside your ear greater. This forces the eardrum to bulge outward. When you swallow or yawn, it releases the pressure. Your eardrum "pops" as it goes back to its normal shape.

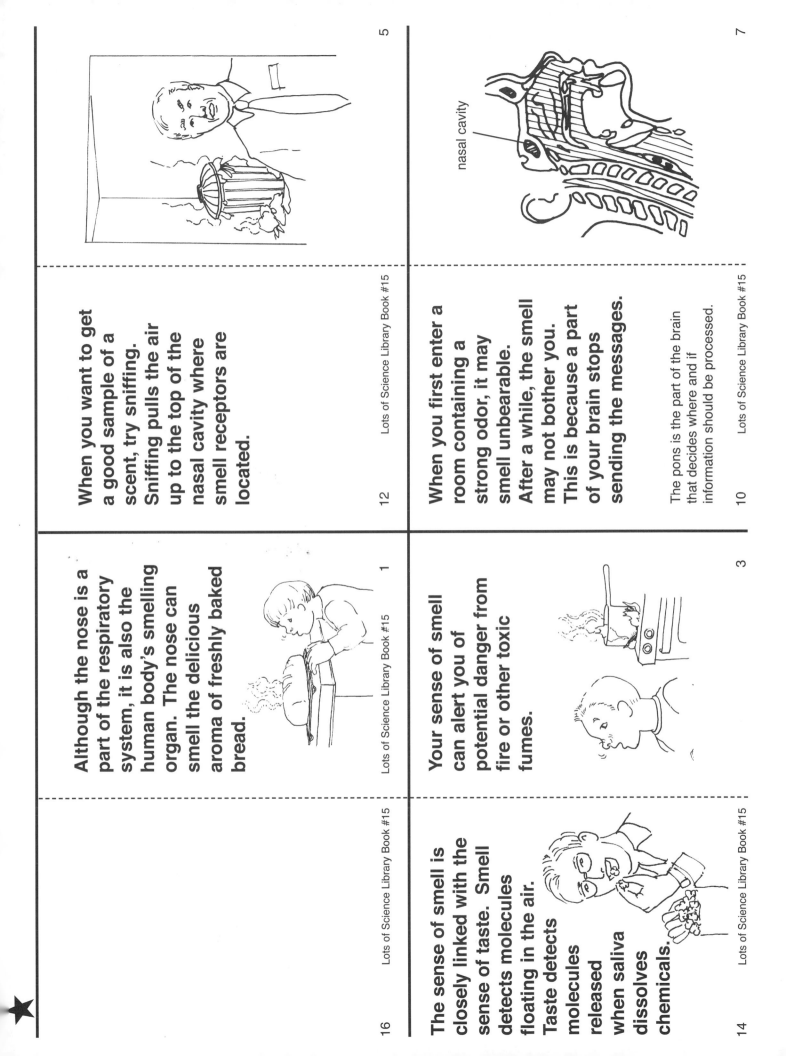

nasal cavity

When you want to get a good sample of a scent, try sniffing. Sniffing pulls the air up to the top of the nasal cavity where smell receptors are located.

12

When you first enter a room containing a strong odor, it may smell unbearable. After a while, the smell may not bother you. This is because a part of your brain stops sending the messages.

The pons is the part of the brain that decides where and if information should be processed.

10

Although the nose is a part of the respiratory system, it is also the human body's smelling organ. The nose can smell the delicious aroma of freshly baked bread.

1

Your sense of smell can alert you of potential danger from fire or other toxic fumes.

3

16

The sense of smell is closely linked with the sense of taste. Smell detects molecules floating in the air. Taste detects molecules released when saliva dissolves chemicals.

14

Signals are sent from the olfactory bulb to the brain through the olfactory nerve.

Nerves connected to these receptors send odor information to the olfactory bulb, the "smell factory." From the olfactory bulb, signals are sent to the brain.

Inside the nasal cavity, air is cleaned and warmed. Special feelers, or smell receptors, on the roof of the nasal cavity pick up smells as they pass through the nose.

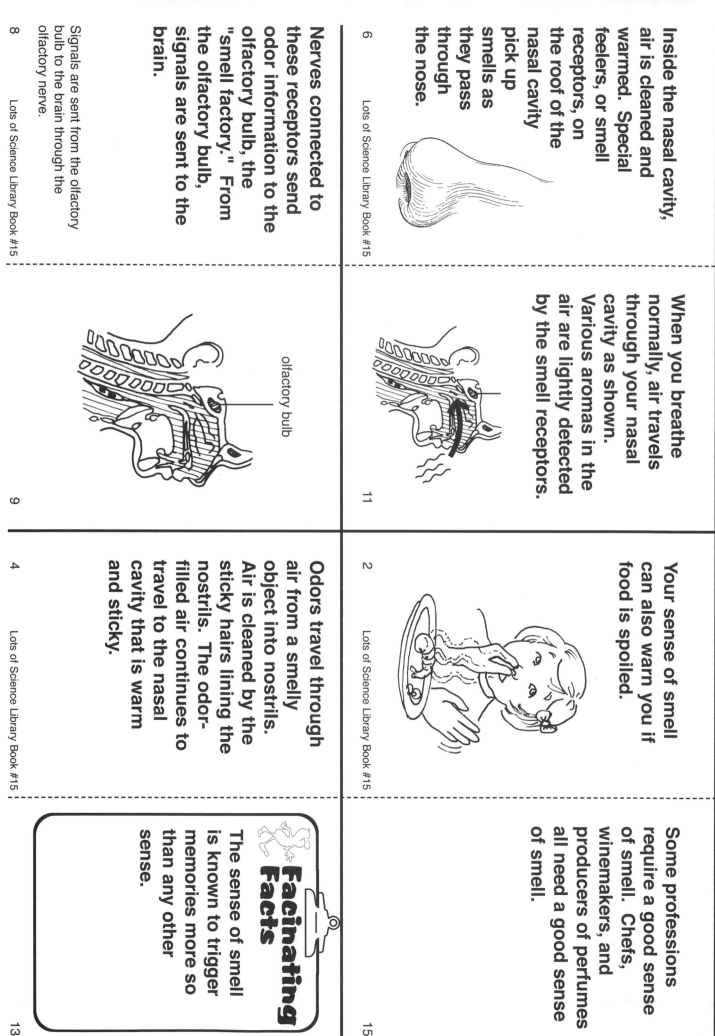

olfactory bulb

When you breathe normally, air travels through your nasal cavity as shown. Various aromas in the air are lightly detected by the smell receptors.

Signals are sent from the olfactory bulb to the brain through the olfactory nerve.

Odors travel through air from a smelly object into nostrils. Air is cleaned by the sticky hairs lining the nostrils. The odor-filled air continues to travel to the nasal cavity that is warm and sticky.

Your sense of smell can also warn you if food is spoiled.

Some professions require a good sense of smell. Chefs, winemakers, and producers of perfumes all need a good sense of smell.

Facinating Facts

The sense of smell is known to trigger memories more so than any other sense.

Taste buds located in various sections on the tongue distinguish four main flavors: **sweet, sour, salty, and bitter.**

sour
salty

bitter
sour
salty
sweet

Facinating Facts

Young children have more taste buds than adults on their tongue and lips.

Look at your tongue and you will see that it is covered with small and larger bumps. These bumps help your tongue grip food.

The bumps on the tongue are called papillae. The small bumps are called filiform papillae; the larger bumps are called fungiform papillae.

After you smell freshly baked bread, you may want to eat it. The smell and taste of the delicious bread are difficult to separate. This is because your sense of taste is largely connected to your sense of smell.

---

salivary glands

Sour tastes are detected by the taste buds located on the sides of the tongue. Finally, bitter flavors are located at the back of the tongue.

Taste buds located at the tip of the tongue detect sweet flavors.

When you have a cold and cannot smell, food doesn't taste as good. Along with smell, the sensation of taste is also factored by the food's texture, temperature, and appearance.

The tongue is a large muscle and the human body's main organ of taste. After you bite into an apple, saliva moistens and dissolves the chemicals in the food. Your tongue helps you move the food around as you chew.

Your nose detects odors by smelling molecules floating in the air. Your sense of taste occurs when food enters your mouth and is moistened by saliva. Saliva is a special liquid excreted in your mouth to help moisten food and begin the digestion process.

The sense of taste makes eating an enjoyable experience. Taste also serves a safety purpose. If you did not have a sense of taste, you could eat spoiled food and get sick.

The tongue consists of about 10,000 taste buds, located on the surface of the tongue.

On the sides of the tip of the tongue are taste buds that sense salty flavors.

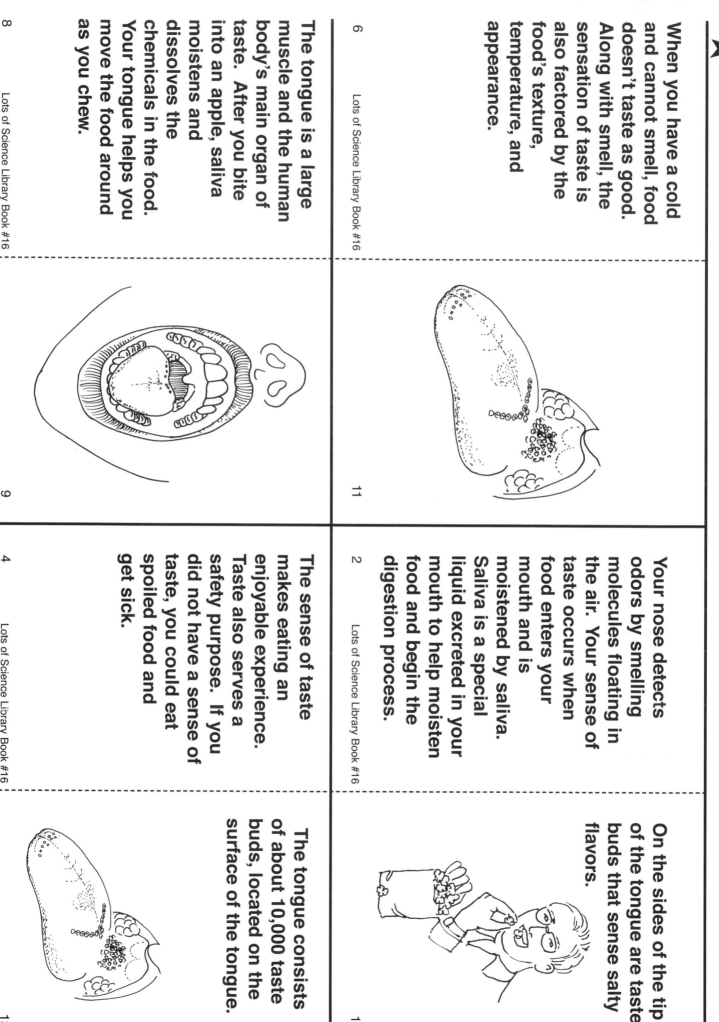

Under the surface of your skin are special organs called receptors. Receptors are part of the nervous system and help process sensations of pain, temperature, and pressure. Touch receptors are found in the epidermis and dermis.

When a feather lands on your arm, you feel it because light touch receptors are located just below the epidermis. These receptors are located mostly on the body where there is little or no hair.

Goose bumps are formed when your body is cold because the blood vessels move into your skin to prevent heat loss. Tiny muscles next to each hair follicle contract. The contraction pulls the follicles upright and makes the hairs stand up.

Pressure receptors are located deep within the skin, or the dermis. The palms of your hands and the soles of your feet contain many pressure receptors.

cold receptor

hair root pressure receptor

heat receptor

pressure receptors

touch receptors

When you pet a kitten, you feel its soft fur, its warmth, and the vibrations of its purring. Your sense of touch has given you a pleasurable experience.

Although you may think that it would be nice to not feel pain, the feeling of pain can protect you from many dangers. If you could not feel heat or pain when you touched something hot, you would be burned.

Touch receptors are not evenly distributed throughout the human body. Large amounts of receptors are located in the fingertips, toes, lips, and tongue. The middle of the back has the fewest receptors.

Pain and heat receptors are called free nerve endings.

Pain and heat receptors are also located near the skin's surface. Receptors send electrical signals to the brain.

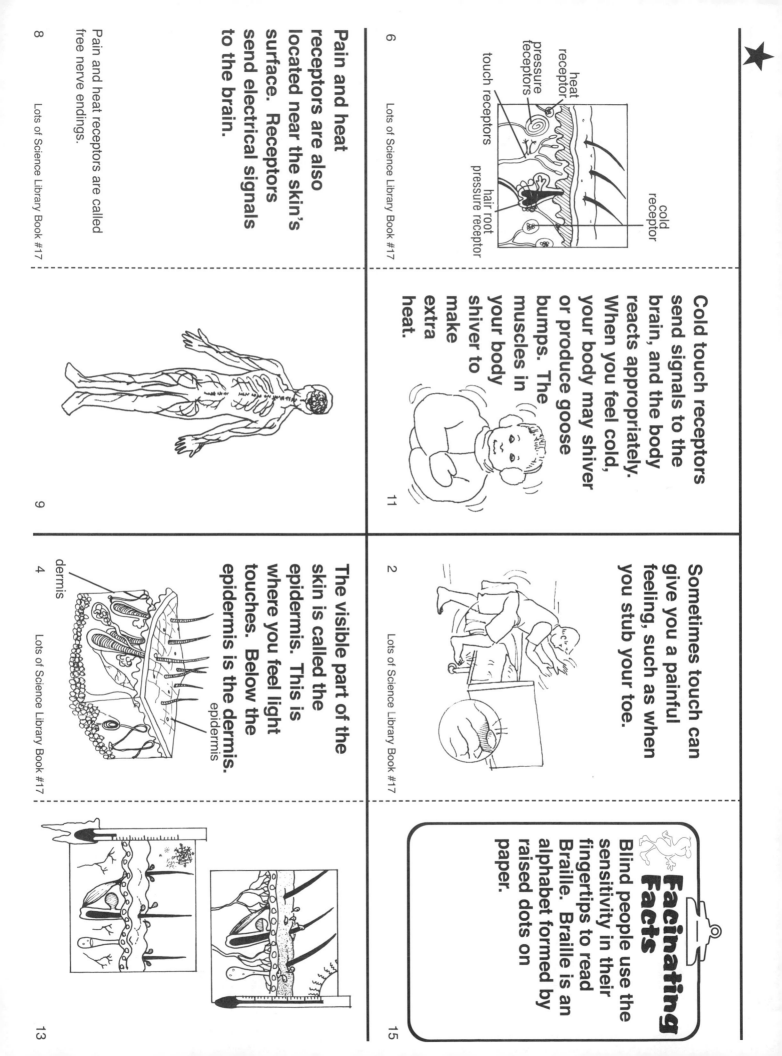

heat receptor

pressure receptors

touch receptors

cold receptor

hair root

pressure receptor

Cold touch receptors send signals to the brain, and the body reacts appropriately. When you feel cold, your body may shiver or produce goose bumps. The muscles in your body shiver to make extra heat.

The visible part of the skin is called the epidermis. This is where you feel light touches. Below the epidermis is the dermis.

dermis

epidermis

Sometimes touch can give you a painful feeling, such as when you stub your toe.

Facinating Facts

Blind people use the sensitivity in their fingertips to read Braille. Braille is an alphabet formed by raised dots on paper.

Saliva is produced in the salivary glands. They are located under the tongue and around the jaw. The salivary glands are called parotid glands, submandibular glands, and sublingual glands.

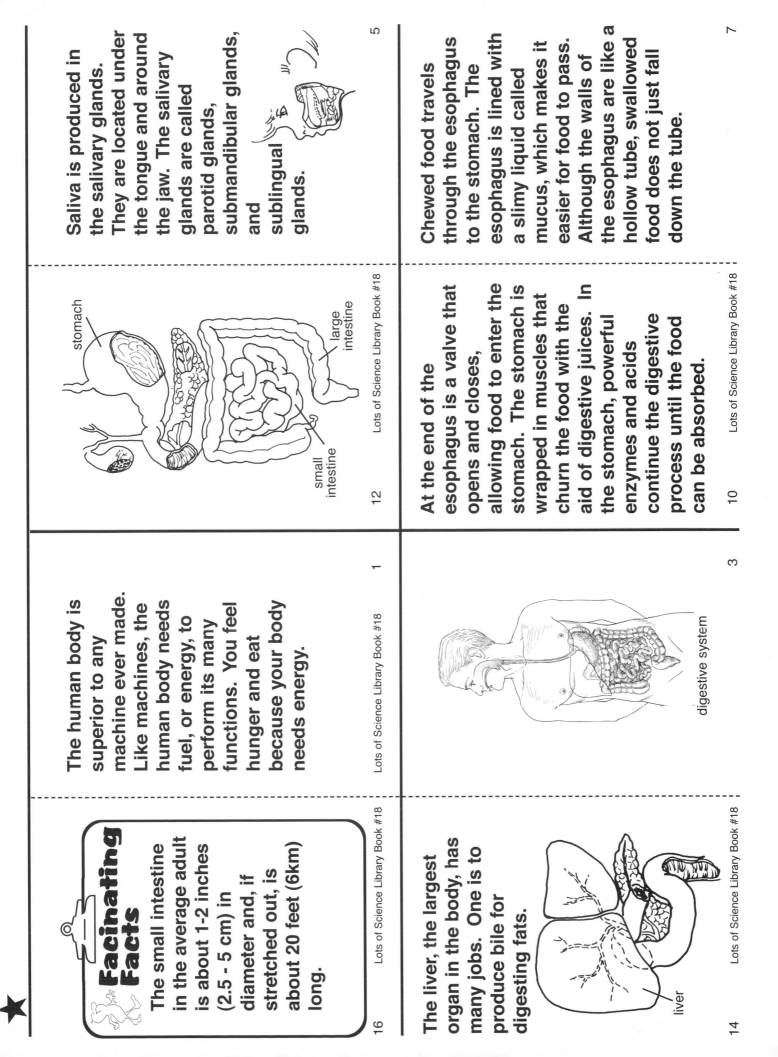

stomach

small intestine

large intestine

Chewed food travels through the esophagus to the stomach. The esophagus is lined with a slimy liquid called mucus, which makes it easier for food to pass. Although the walls of the esophagus are like a hollow tube, swallowed food does not just fall down the tube.

At the end of the esophagus is a valve that opens and closes, allowing food to enter the stomach. The stomach is wrapped in muscles that churn the food with the aid of digestive juices. In the stomach, powerful enzymes and acids continue the digestive process until the food can be absorbed.

The human body is superior to any machine ever made. Like machines, the human body needs fuel, or energy, to perform its many functions. You feel hunger and eat because your body needs energy.

digestive system

Facinating Facts

The small intestine in the average adult is about 1-2 inches (2.5 - 5 cm) in diameter and, if stretched out, is about 20 feet (6km) long.

The liver, the largest organ in the body, has many jobs. One is to produce bile for digesting fats.

liver

As the food softens, your tongue moves it to the back of the mouth. When you swallow food, your nose and windpipe automatically close so that food does not enter your nose and lungs.

The windpipe is called the trachea. The epiglottis blocks the trachea when you swallow food.

The food, now a thick liquid, leaves the stomach and enters the small intestine. The liquid food travels into the small intestine and mixes with the digestive juices from the pancreas and gallbladder. Most absorption occurs in the small intestine where nutrients from digested food are absorbed into the bloodstream.

The walls of the esophagus are lined with muscles that expand and contract to push the food down into the stomach. This is why you can swallow food when you're standing or lying down.

The process of the esophagus muscles expanding and contracting is called peristalsis.

digestive system

Food that enters your mouth is broken down by your digestive system. In the digestive system, food is broken down into tiny particles that can be absorbed into the bloodstream and carried throughout the body.

The remaining food passes into the large intestine where water is removed to be used by the body. Undigested food that cannot be used by the body is expelled or excreted through the anus as waste. This waste is called feces.

Digestion begins in the mouth when you chew food. Teeth grind food, the tongue moves the food around, and a special fluid called saliva helps to break it down. Saliva helps digest food by moistening it, and it contains special substances called enzymes that help break down the food even more.

Absorption occurs through tiny hair-like structures called villi that line the inner walls of the small intestines. Villi absorb food like the fibers of a paper towel.

Waste water, or urine, travels through the right and left ureter into the bladder. The muscular walls of the bladder expand and contract depending on how much urine it is storing. The bladder stores the urine until it is eliminated through the urethra.

Sometimes, when people have a diseased or injured kidneys, an operation is performed to replace a damaged kidney with a healthy one. This is called a kidney transplant. Healthy kidneys may be obtained from a living person who donates one of their two kidneys.

If urea is not eliminated, poisons may cause illness and eventually death. When a person's kidneys cannot function due to injury or disease, they can lead a fairly normal life by using a dialysis machine.

As you have learned, blood leaves the heart and travels throughout the body nourishing all body cells. The used blood contains waste products that must be eliminated. The urinary system filters waste from the blood and expels it.

kidney
ureter
urethra
kidney
ureter
bladder

Doctors often examine a patients' urine to help them reach a diagnosis. For example, the presence of various substances can indicate diabetes, infection, cancer, or pregnancy.

Facinating Facts

People can live normal lives with one healthy kidney. If one kidney is removed, the remaining kidney can increase in size by about 50% within a short time.

Bile pigment in urine is called urobilin.

Bile is produced in the liver to help digest fats in food. Urine's yellowish brown color comes from the broken down bile.

Facinating Facts

Kidneys filter a human body's entire blood supply 360 times a day. An average adult eliminates about 3 pints (1.5 L) of urine each day.

The star

A dialysis machine is like an artificial kidney. It removes waste products from the patient's blood. A tube is attached to an artery in the patient's arm and their blood is pumped through a filter in the dialysis machine where it is cleaned and then returned through a vein in the patient's other arm.

The contents of urine depend somewhat on what you have eaten and drunk, but basically urine consists of about 95% water and 5% waste products, including urea. Urea is the by-product produced by your body when energy is burned.

The tiny filtering units in the kidney are called nephrons.

A kidney consists of more than a million microscopic filtering units. Inside the kidneys, blood is continuously being filtered and cleaned and returned to the heart. Clean blood goes back into the bloodstream.

The urinary system consists of two kidneys, two ureters, a bladder, and urethra. The right and left kidneys are located above the waist on each side of the spine. Kidneys are reddish, bean-shaped organs about the size of a bar of soap.

A patient may receive a kidney from an organ donor who has just died. Frequently, people have donor information printed on the back of their driver's license. Kidney transplants are one of the most successful organ transplants.

Kidney transplants using a kidney from a close relative has less potential problems because the tissues of the donor and patient are often similar.

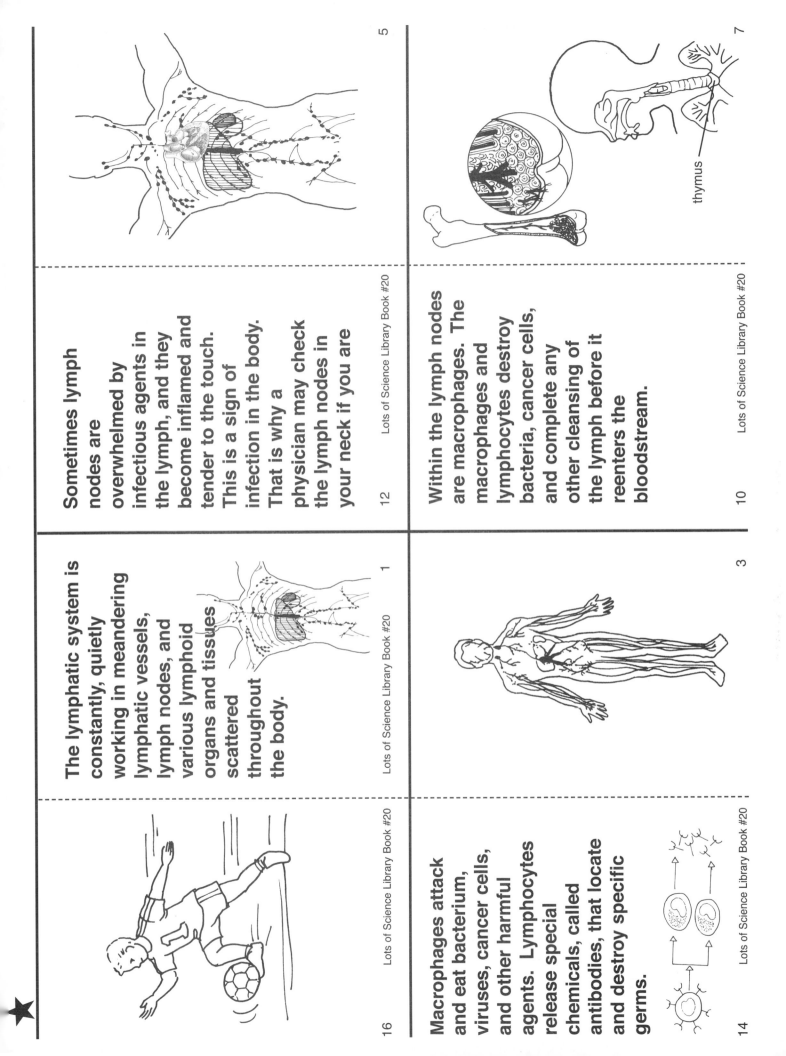

5

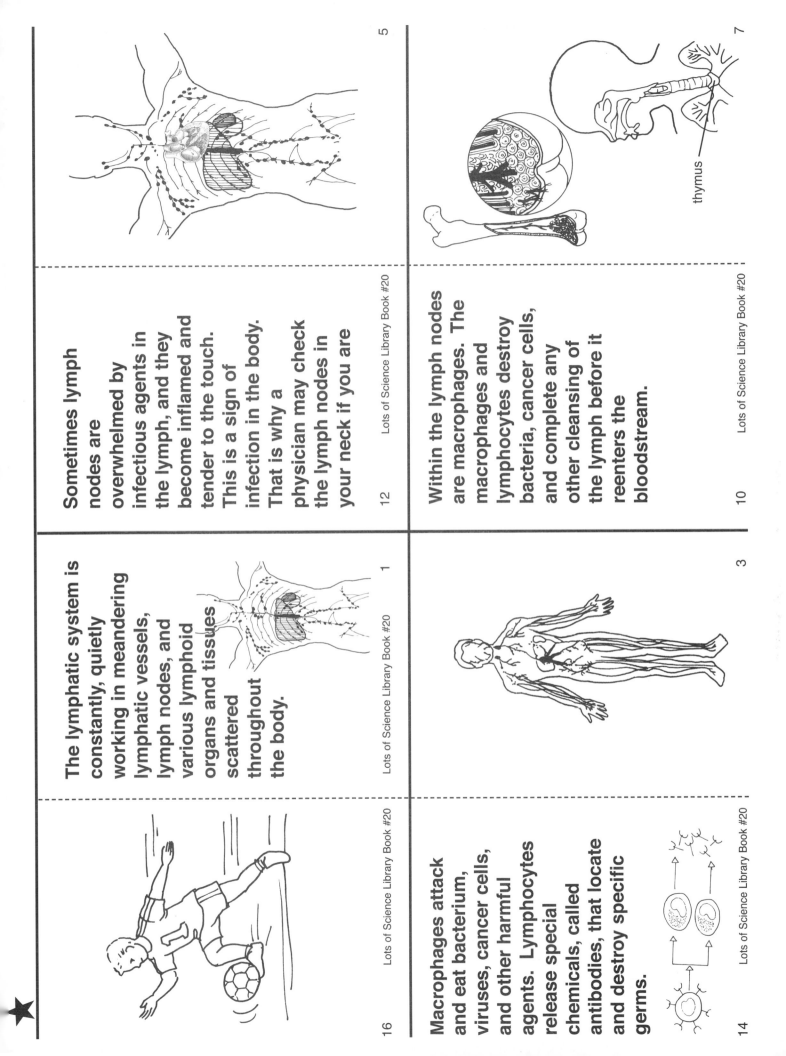

7

Sometimes lymph nodes are overwhelmed by infectious agents in the lymph, and they become inflamed and tender to the touch. This is a sign of infection in the body. That is why a physician may check the lymph nodes in your neck if you are

12

Within the lymph nodes are macrophages. The macrophages and lymphocytes destroy bacteria, cancer cells, and complete any other cleansing of the lymph before it reenters the bloodstream.

10

The lymphatic system is constantly, quietly working in meandering lymphatic vessels, lymph nodes, and various lymphoid organs and tissues scattered throughout the body.

1

3

Macrophages attack and eat bacterium, viruses, cancer cells, and other harmful agents. Lymphocytes release special chemicals, called antibodies, that locate and destroy specific germs.

16

14

★

8

There are hundreds of glands in the human body called lymph nodes. They are usually embedded in tissues and therefore hard to locate. Lymph nodes are most abundant in the neck, armpit, and groin areas.

6

Lymphocytes are cells that fight disease in the bloodstream, organs, and tissues. Lymphocytes are produced in the bone marrow and the thymus.

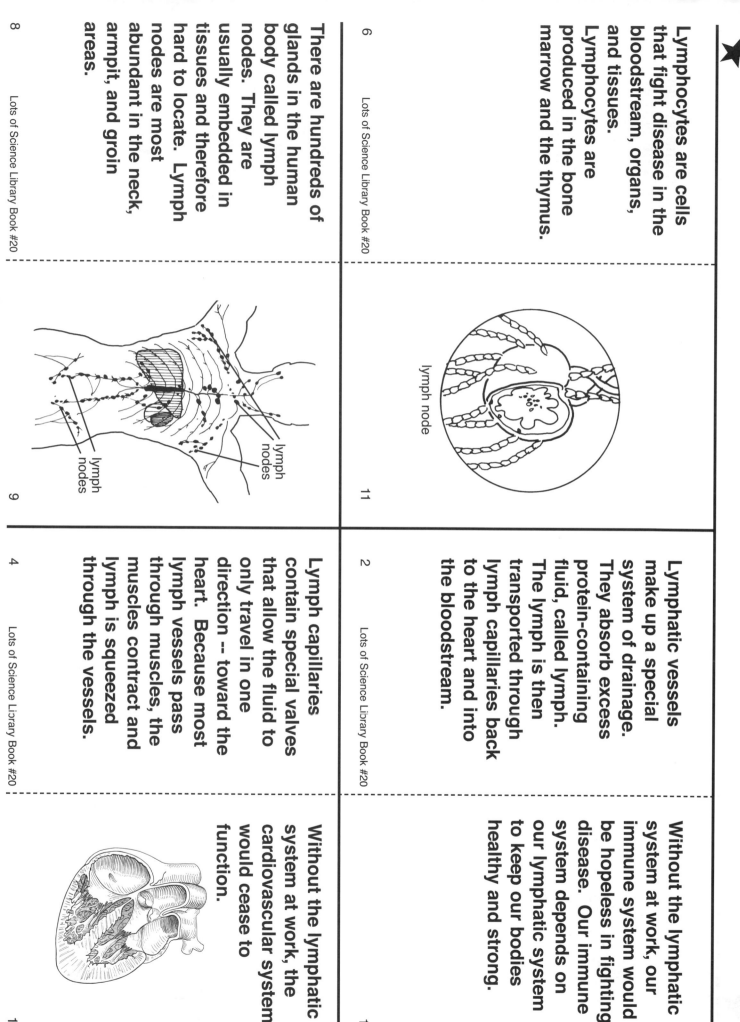

lymph nodes

lymph nodes

9

lymph node

11

4

Lymph capillaries contain special valves that allow the fluid to only travel in one direction -- toward the heart. Because most lymph vessels pass through muscles, the muscles contract and lymph is squeezed through the vessels.

2

Lymphatic vessels make up a special system of drainage. They absorb excess protein-containing fluid, called lymph. The lymph is then transported through lymph capillaries back to the heart and into the bloodstream.

Without the lymphatic system at work, the cardiovascular system would cease to function.

Without the lymphatic system at work, our immune system would be hopeless in fighting disease. Our immune system depends on our lymphatic system to keep our bodies healthy and strong.

15

13

The immune system depends on lymph nodes to destroy bacteria.

---

antigens

This is the body's natural process to becoming immune to certain bacteria or viruses. Today, we have methods of helping the body become immune to specific bacteria or viruses through artificial means.

Antibodies multiply to fight the germs that are also multiplying. When germs are destroyed by antibodies, these same antibodies exist in the body, ready to attack the antigen if it returns in the future. The body is now immune to this antigen.

The human body is constantly under attack from germs such as bacteria and viruses. These germs, are in air, water, food, and in and on your body. If these germs are allowed to multiply in the body, illness or disease may result.

Disease-causing germs are called pathogens.

The first line of defense is the skin. The skin protects the body from outside germs.

Later, if this person is invaded by the original disease-causing germ, lymphocytes will recognize it and produce antibodies to destroy it.

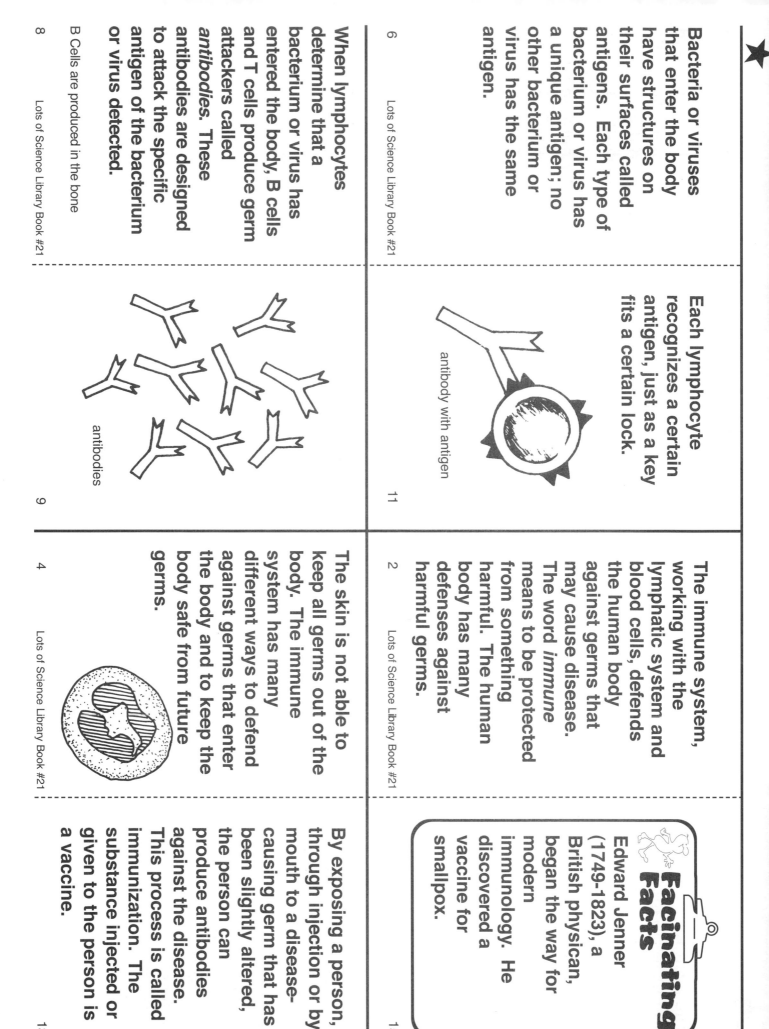

2

The immune system, working with the lymphatic system and blood cells, defends the human body against germs that may cause disease. The word *immune* means to be protected from something harmful. The human body has many defenses against harmful germs.

Lots of Science Library Book #21

4

The skin is not able to keep all germs out of the body. The immune system has many different ways to defend against germs that enter the body and to keep the body safe from future germs.

6

Bacteria or viruses that enter the body have structures on their surfaces called antigens. Each type of bacterium or virus has a unique antigen; no other bacterium or virus has the same antigen.

Lots of Science Library Book #21

8

When lymphocytes determine that a bacterium or virus has entered the body, B cells and T cells produce germ attackers called *antibodies*. These antibodies are designed to attack the specific antigen of the bacterium or virus detected.

B Cells are produced in the bone

9

antibodies

11

Each lymphocyte recognizes a certain antigen, just as a key fits a certain lock.

antibody with antigen

13

By exposing a person, through injection or by mouth to a disease-causing germ that has been slightly altered, the person can produce antibodies against the disease. This process is called immunization. The substance injected or given to the person is a vaccine.

15

Facinating Facts

Edward Jenner (1749-1823), a British physican, began the way for modern immunology. He discovered a vaccine for smallpox.

The pituitary gland and the hypothalamus are located in the brain. The pituitary gland, the master gland, controls all other hormone-producing glands.

hypothalamus

pituitary

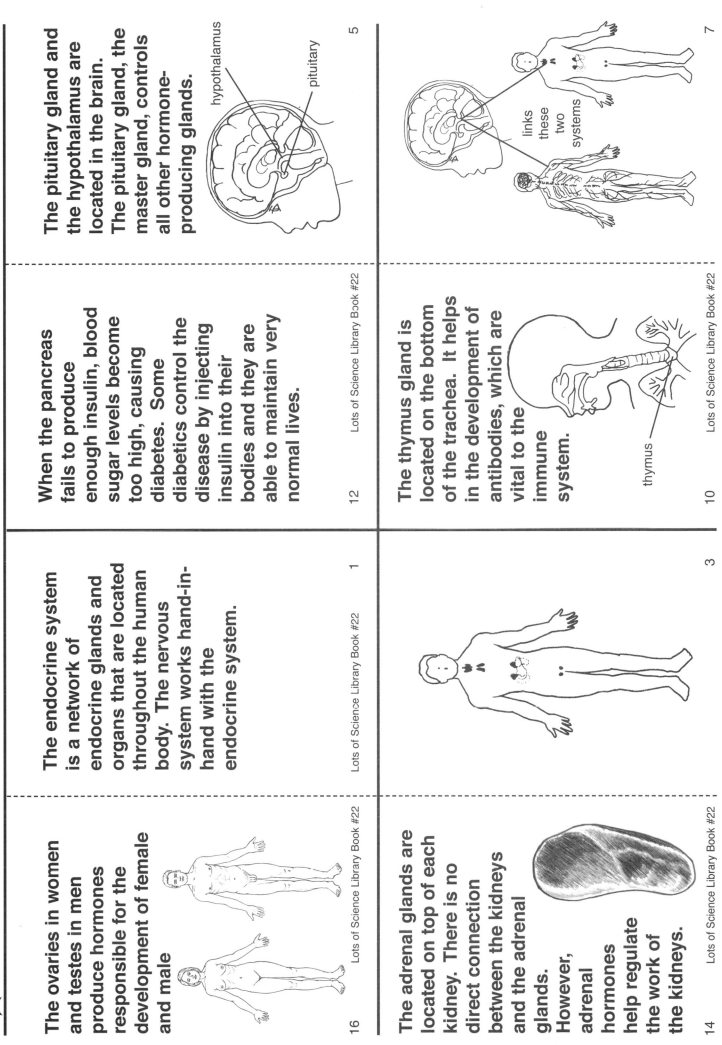

links these two systems

When the pancreas fails to produce enough insulin, blood sugar levels become too high, causing diabetes. Some diabetics control the disease by injecting insulin into their bodies and they are able to maintain very normal lives.

The thymus gland is located on the bottom of the trachea. It helps in the development of antibodies, which are vital to the immune system.

thymus

The endocrine system is a network of endocrine glands and organs that are located throughout the human body. The nervous system works hand-in-hand with the endocrine system.

The ovaries in women and testes in men produce hormones responsible for the development of female and male

The adrenal glands are located on top of each kidney. There is no direct connection between the kidneys and the adrenal glands. However, adrenal hormones help regulate the work of the kidneys.

★

Growth hormones are produced in the pituitary gland. The pituitary gland also controls kidney function and regulates blood pressure. The hypothalamus links the endocrine system with the nervous system.

The pancreas, located behind the stomach, produces powerful juices that aid in digestion. Insulin, the hormone that controls the sugar level in blood, is produced in the pancreas. The pancreas also allows the liver to store sugar.

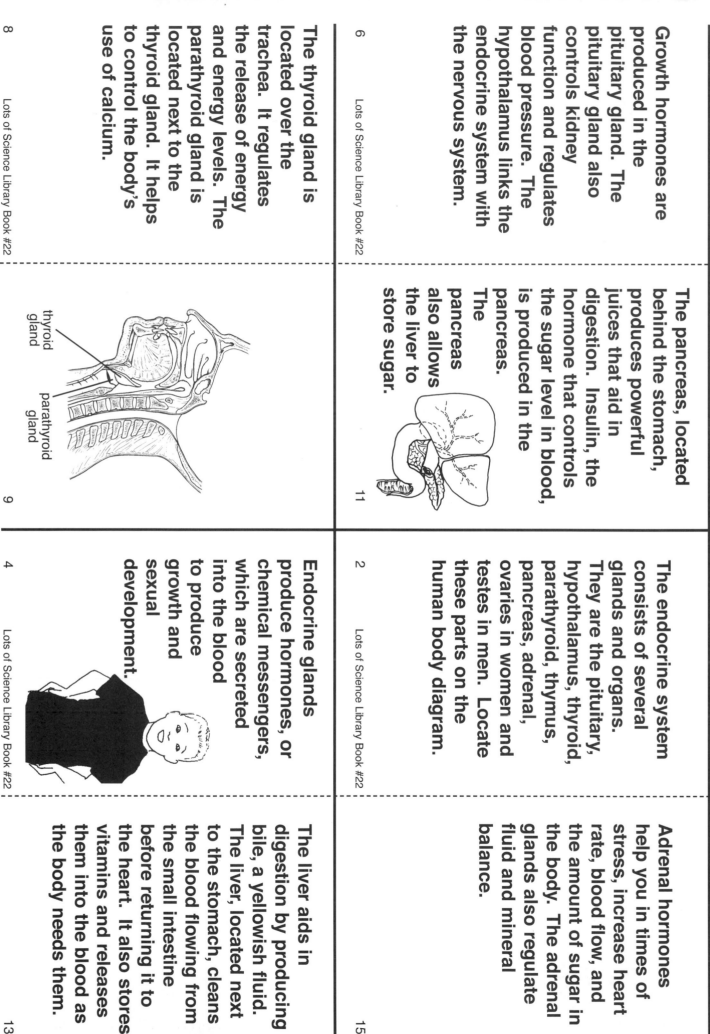

The thyroid gland is located over the trachea. It regulates the release of energy and energy levels. The parathyroid gland is located next to the thyroid gland. It helps to control the body's use of calcium.

thyroid gland

parathyroid gland

The endocrine system consists of several glands and organs. They are the pituitary, hypothalamus, thyroid, parathyroid, thymus, pancreas, adrenal, ovaries in women and testes in men. Locate these parts on the human body diagram.

Adrenal hormones help you in times of stress, increase heart rate, blood flow, and the amount of sugar in the body. The adrenal glands also regulate fluid and mineral balance.

Endocrine glands produce hormones, or chemical messengers, which are secreted into the blood to produce growth and sexual development.

The liver aids in digestion by producing bile, a yellowish fluid. The liver, located next to the stomach, cleans the blood flowing from the small intestine before returning it to the heart. It also stores vitamins and releases them into the blood as the body needs them.

egg (female sex cell)

sperm (male sex cell)

fallopian Tubes

ovaries

uterus

vagina

Sperm are much smaller than a woman's egg. They are about .002 inches (.05 mm) long. Sperm have a flat, oval head and a tail that whips from side to side to move them forward. They are streamlined to make movement through liquids easier.

A man's reproductive system consists of a penis, testes, and urethra. When a young man reaches puberty, his two testes produce and store male sex cells, called sperm. A sperm duct runs from the testes to the penis through the urethra.

The human body, as marvelous as it is, does not live forever. Life continues because men and women reproduce, or have babies. Although the reproductive systems of men and women are different from one another, they work together to create new life.

Reproductive systems, do not become active until the early to mid-teen years, called puberty. Girls reach puberty around 12 years of age and boys around 14.

After fertilization he embryo continues to grow in the woman's uterus for about nine months.

If an egg is in the fallopian tube and a sperm reaches it, the two join together. This process is called fertilization. Immediately, the fertilized egg begins to divide. The fertilized egg continues to travel through the fallopian tube and it attaches to the lining of the uterus.

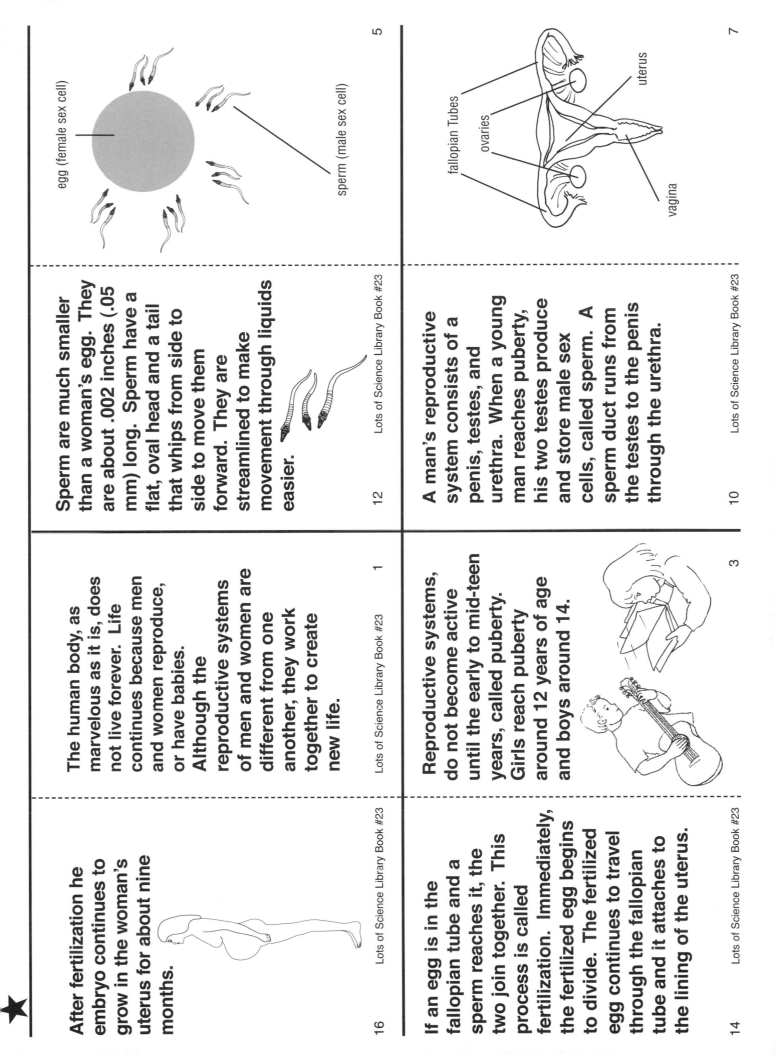

A woman's reproductive system consists of ovaries, fallopian tubes, a uterus, and a vagina. Two ovaries produce, store, and release eggs. When a young girl reaches puberty, her ovaries release one egg every month into a fallopian tube.

The female sex cell is called an ovum. (Plural – ova)

6

A woman's egg is a single cell. It is the only cell that can be seen without a microscope. It is about the size of a pinhead. Once a month an egg is released by an ovary and moves through the fallopian tube to the uterus.

8

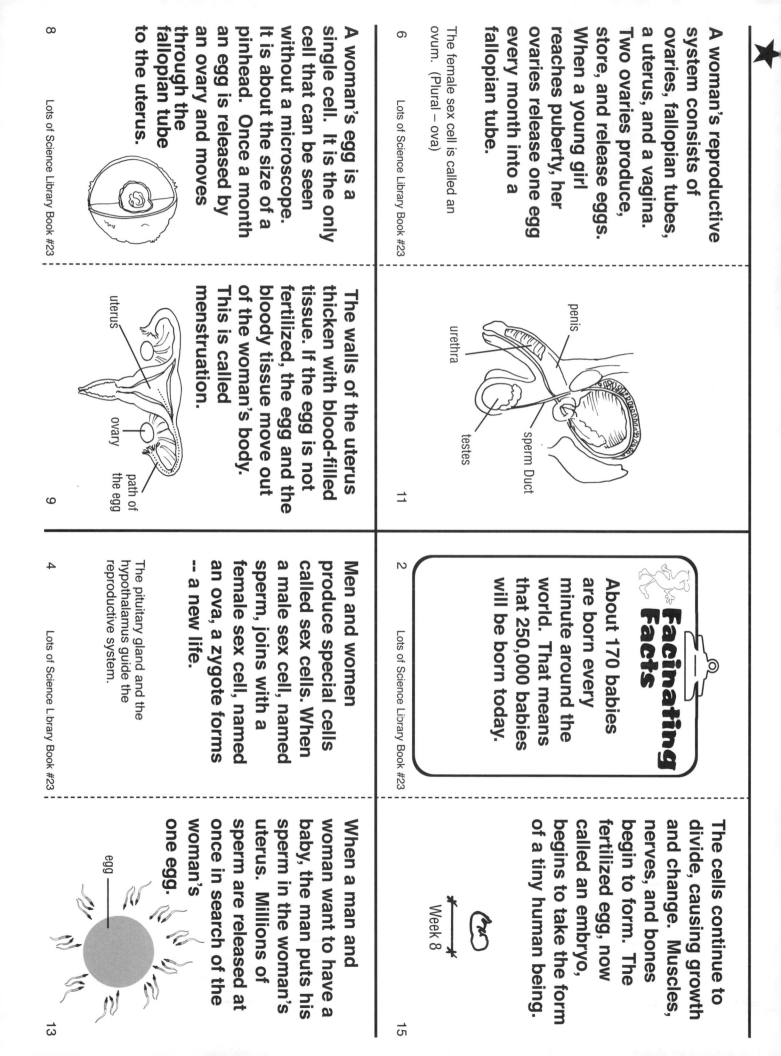

The walls of the uterus thicken with blood-filled tissue. If the egg is not fertilized, the egg and the bloody tissue move out of the woman's body. This is called menstruation.

uterus

ovary

path of the egg

9

penis

urethra

testes

sperm Duct

11

2

Facinating Facts

About 170 babies are born every minute around the world. That means that 250,000 babies will be born today.

Men and women produce special cells called sex cells. When a male sex cell, named sperm, joins with a female sex cell, named an ova, a zygote forms -- a new life.

The pituitary gland and the hypothalamus guide the reproductive system.

4

The cells continue to divide, causing growth and change. Muscles, nerves, and bones begin to form. The fertilized egg, now called an embryo, begins to take the form of a tiny human being.

Week 8

When a man and woman want to have a baby, the man puts his sperm in the woman's uterus. Millions of sperm are released at once in search of the woman's one egg.

egg

15

13

The human body contains systems, organs, and tissues that are all made up of cells. The control center of every cell is the nucleus.

nucleus

Each chromosome consists of about 100,000 genes. Genes are the main structures that determine hereditary traits. A gene is made up of DNA, the molecules that carry hereditary information.

Each sperm and egg contain 23 chromosomes. During fertilization, the sperm and egg join, resulting in 46 chromosomes. If the sperm contains an X-chromosome, the baby will have two X-chromosomes and will be a girl. A girl has received an X-chromosome from her mother and another X-chromosome from her father.

XX

From about the third week, a human form begins to develop and is called an embryo. By now, the placenta, umbilical cord, and amniotic sac have begun to form. The placenta supplies the embryo with nutrients and carries away wastes. The nervous system is rapidly developing and the heart is beating.

The baby is now called a fetus. The fetus grows rapidly during this stage. By 12 weeks, the fetus is about 3 inches (8 cm) long. Sex organs appear, so it is possible to determine the baby's sex at this time.

12 weeks

By 20 weeks, the fetus sleeps, can hear sounds, is about 12-14 inches long, and weighs about 1 pound.

20 weeks

At about 38 weeks, the baby is ready to be born and meet his/her happy parents. On average newborn babies are about 20 inches long and weigh between 7 and 8 pounds.

When a single fertilized egg splits after fertilization, identical twins result. Identical twins share the same placenta, are always the same sex, look the same, and share many similar traits.

Identical twins a   mo

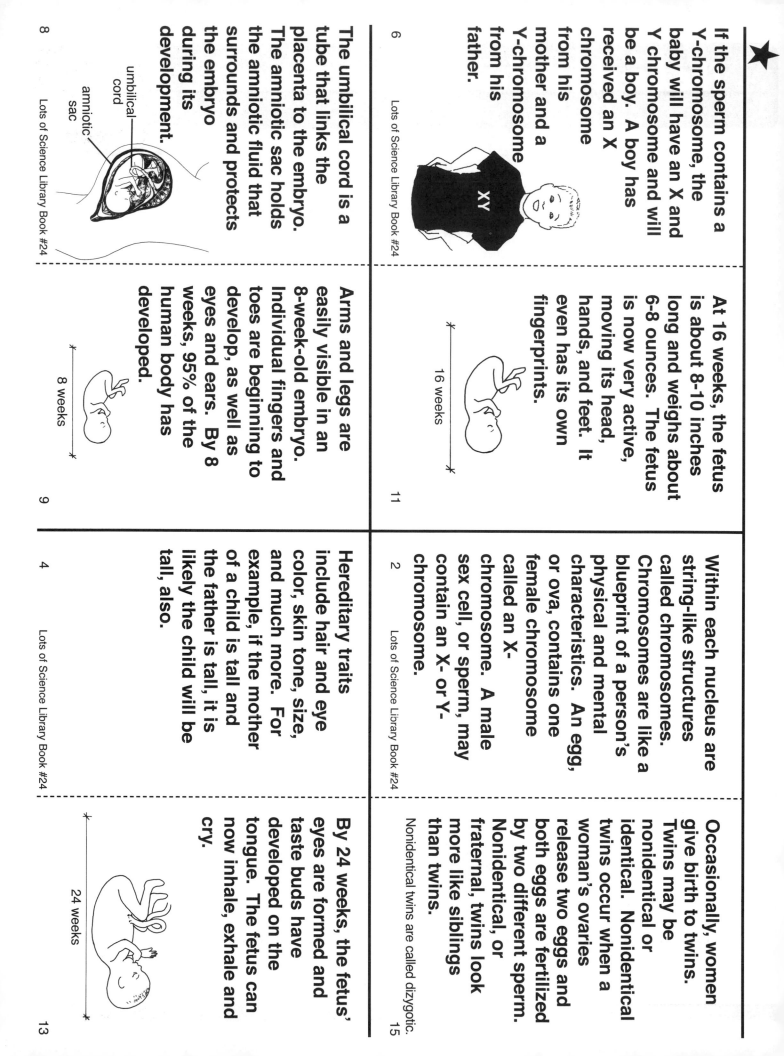

Card (page 6):

If the sperm contains a Y-chromosome, the baby will have an X and Y chromosome and will be a boy. A boy has received an X chromosome from his mother and a Y-chromosome from his father.

XY

Card (page 11):

At 16 weeks, the fetus is about 8-10 inches long and weighs about 6-8 ounces. The fetus is now very active, moving its head, hands, and feet. It even has its own fingerprints.

16 weeks

Card (page 15):

Within each nucleus are string-like structures called chromosomes. Chromosomes are like a blueprint of a person's physical and mental characteristics. An egg, or ova, contains one female chromosome called an X-chromosome. A male sex cell, or sperm, may contain an X- or Y-chromosome.

Occasionally, women give birth to twins. Twins may be nonidentical or identical. Nonidentical twins occur when a woman's ovaries release two eggs and both eggs are fertilized by two different sperm. Nonidentical, or fraternal, twins look more like siblings than twins.

Nonidentical twins are called dizygotic.

Card (page 8):

The umbilical cord is a tube that links the placenta to the embryo. The amniotic sac holds the amniotic fluid that surrounds and protects the embryo during its development.

umbilical cord
amniotic sac

Card (page 9):

Arms and legs are easily visible in an 8-week-old embryo. Individual fingers and toes are beginning to develop, as well as eyes and ears. By 8 weeks, 95% of the human body has developed.

8 weeks

Card (page 2):

Hereditary traits include hair and eye color, skin tone, size, and much more. For example, if the mother of a child is tall and the father is tall, it is likely the child will be tall, also.

Card (page 13):

By 24 weeks, the fetus' eyes are formed and taste buds have developed on the tongue. The fetus can now inhale, exhale and cry.

24 weeks

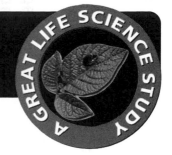
Graphics Pages

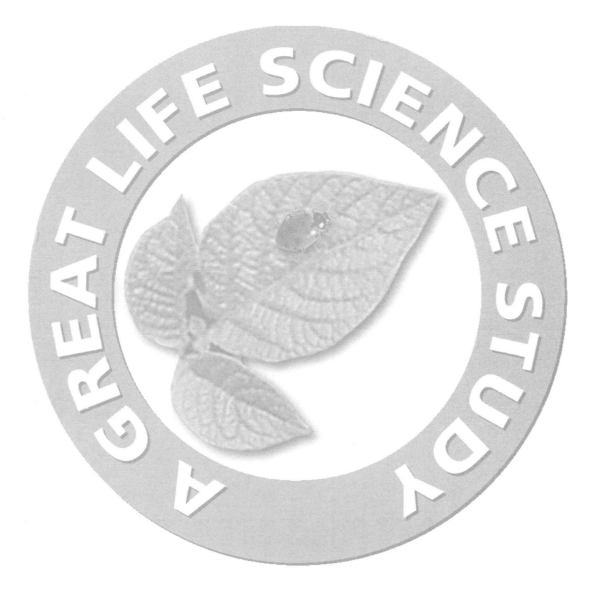

Investigative Loop™

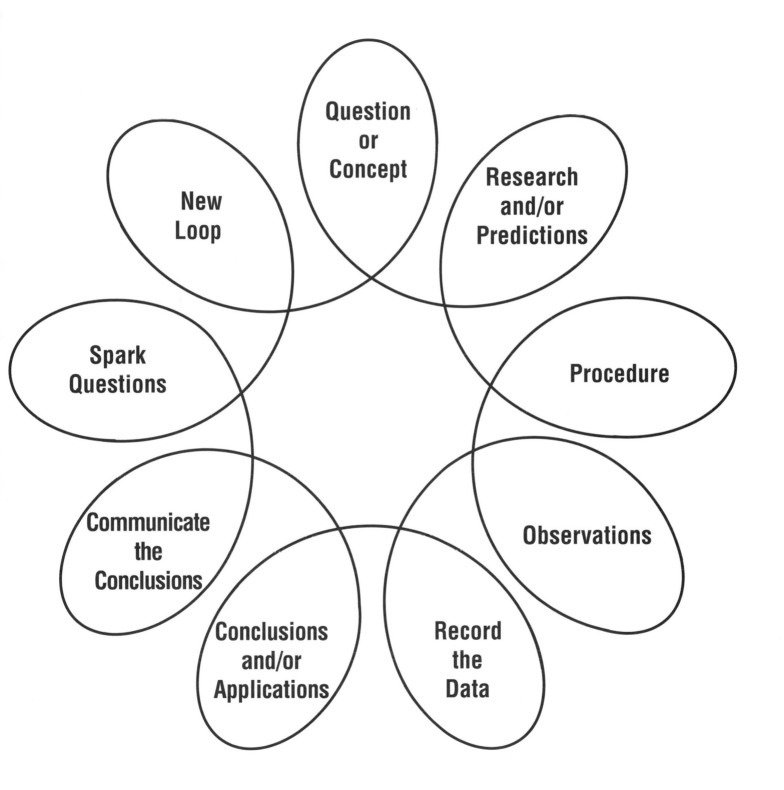

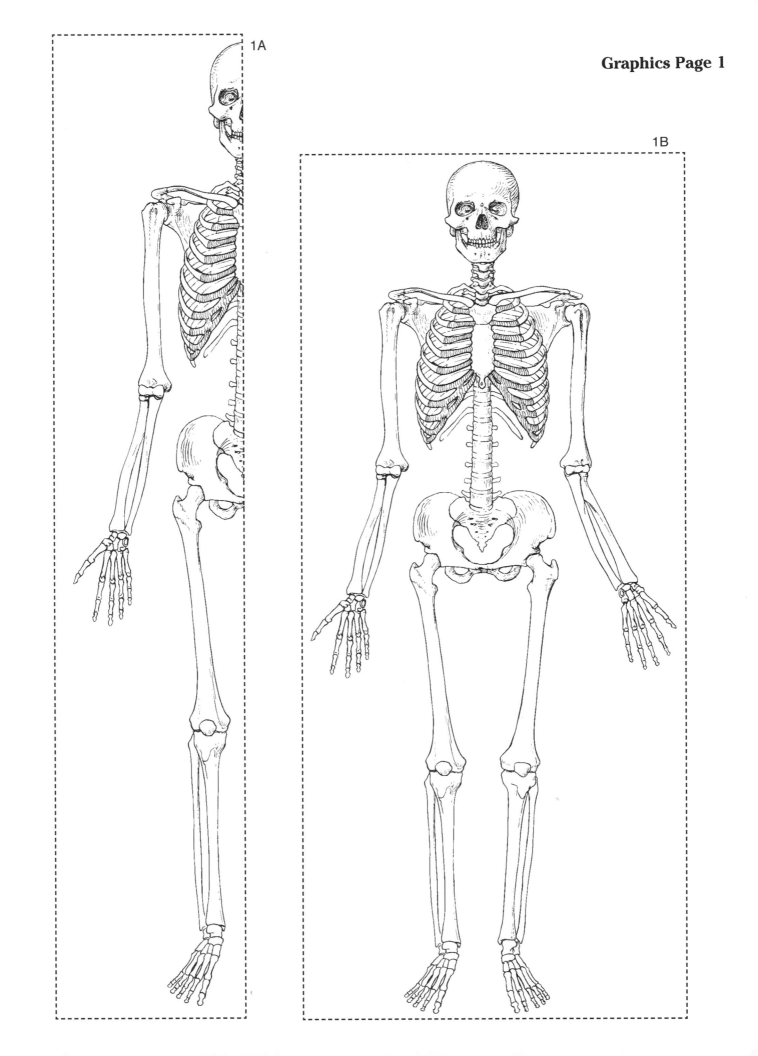

1A

1B

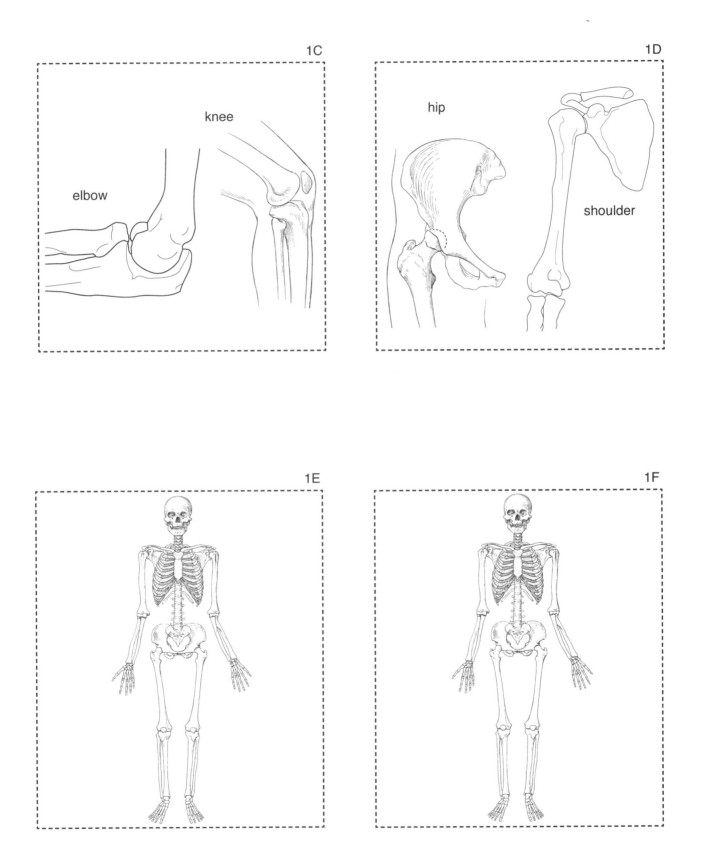

1C

elbow

knee

1D

hip

shoulder

1E

1F

2A

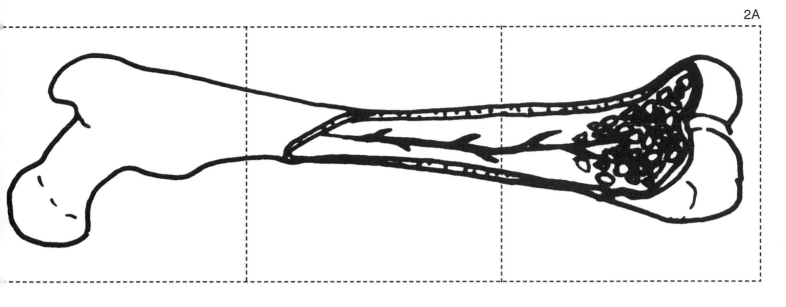

2B

2C

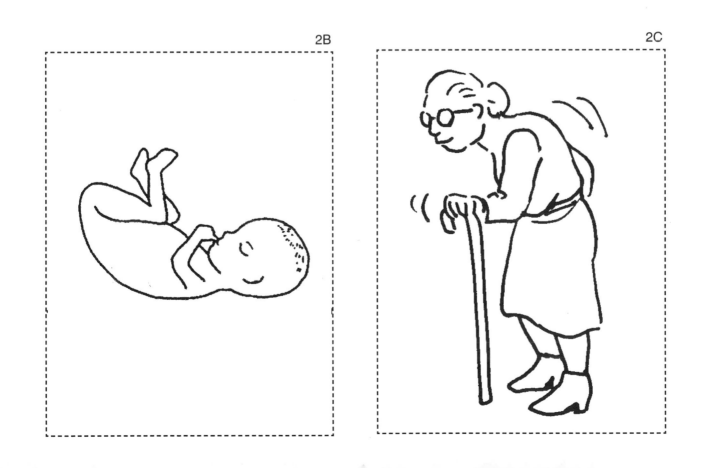

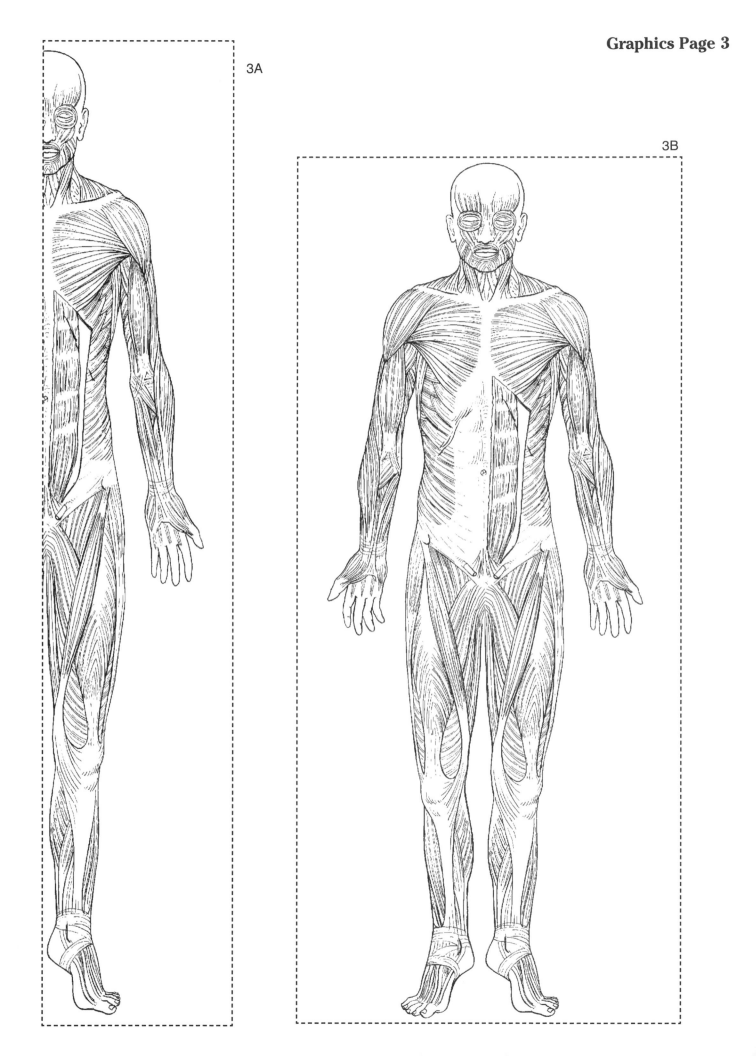

3A

3B

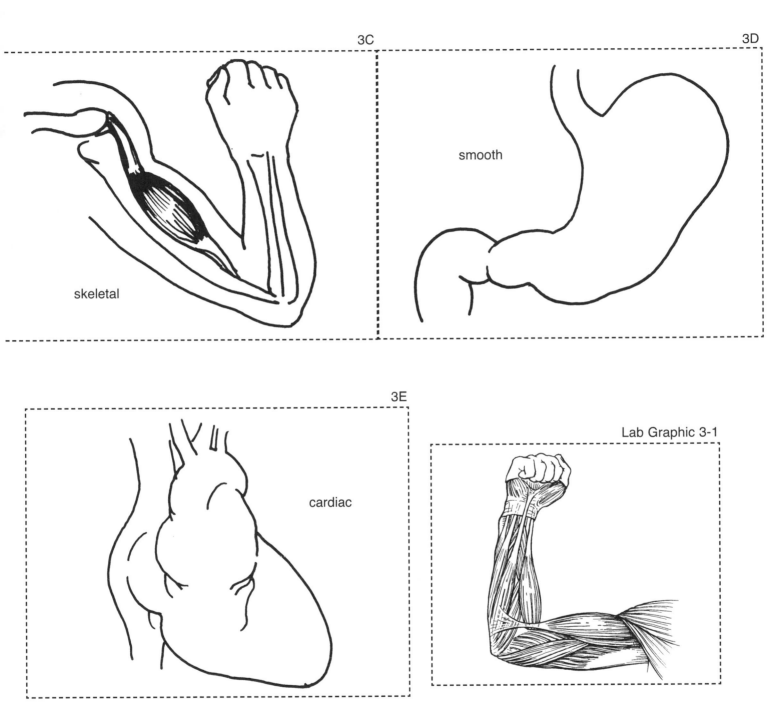

3C

skeletal

3D

smooth

3E

cardiac

Lab Graphic 3-1

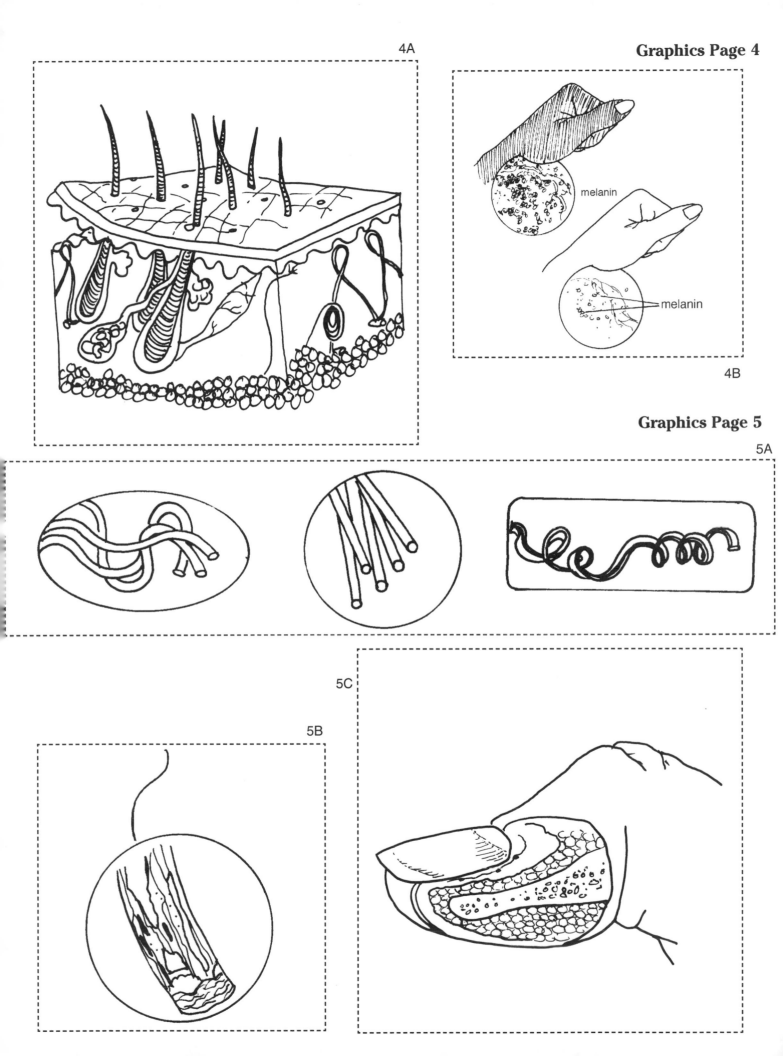

4A

melanin

melanin

4B

5A

5C

5B

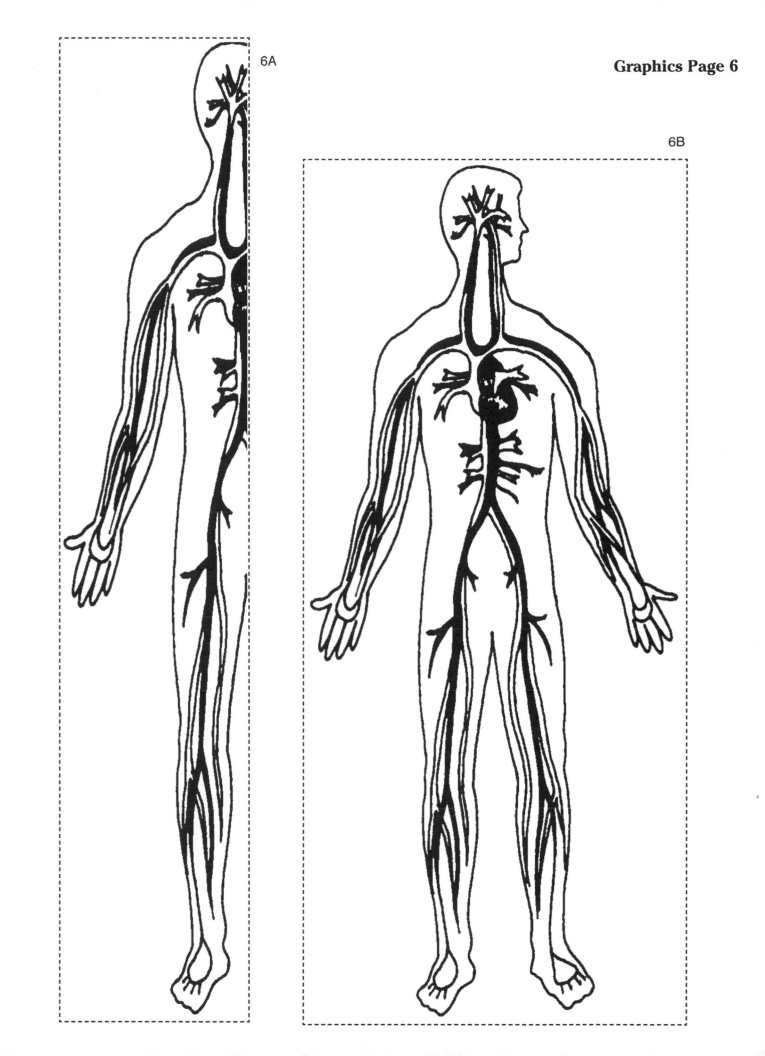

6A

6B

6C   6D   6E   6F

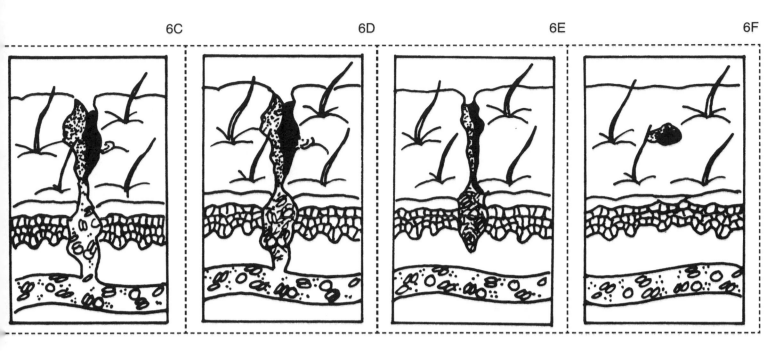

7A

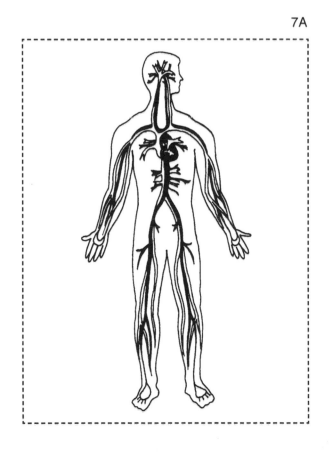

7B

7C

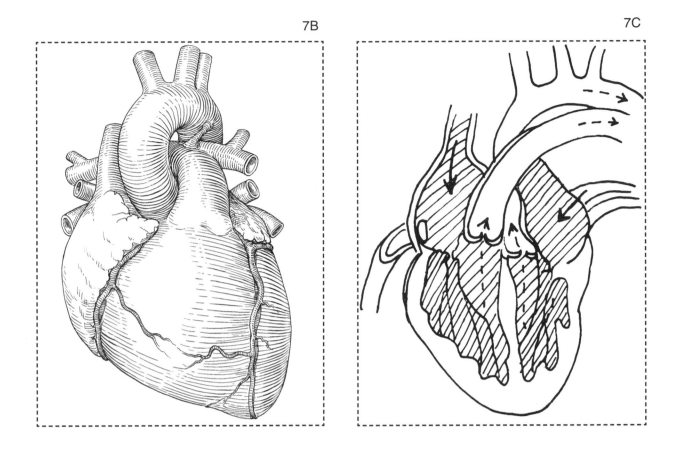

Lab Graphic 7-1

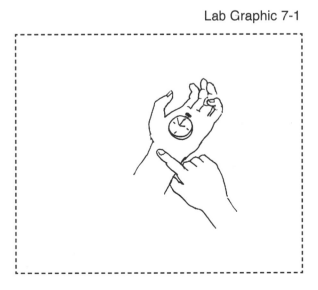

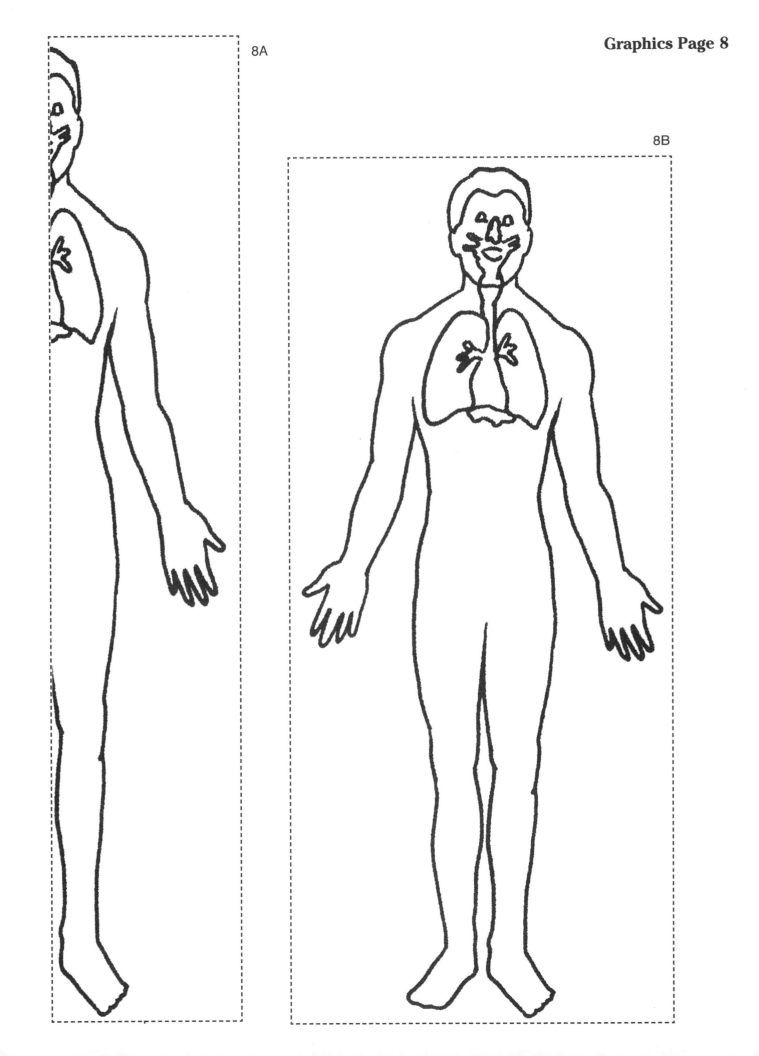

8A

8B

8C

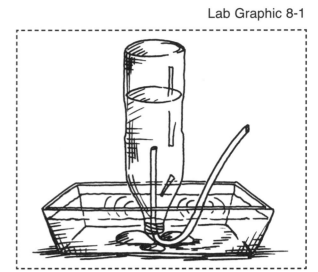

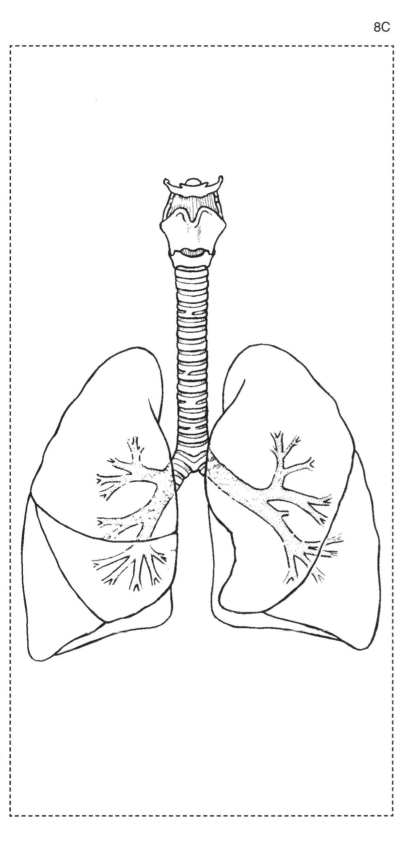

9A

9B

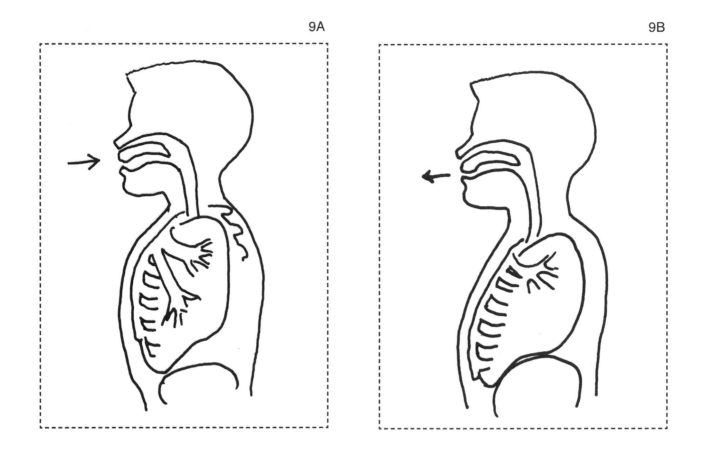

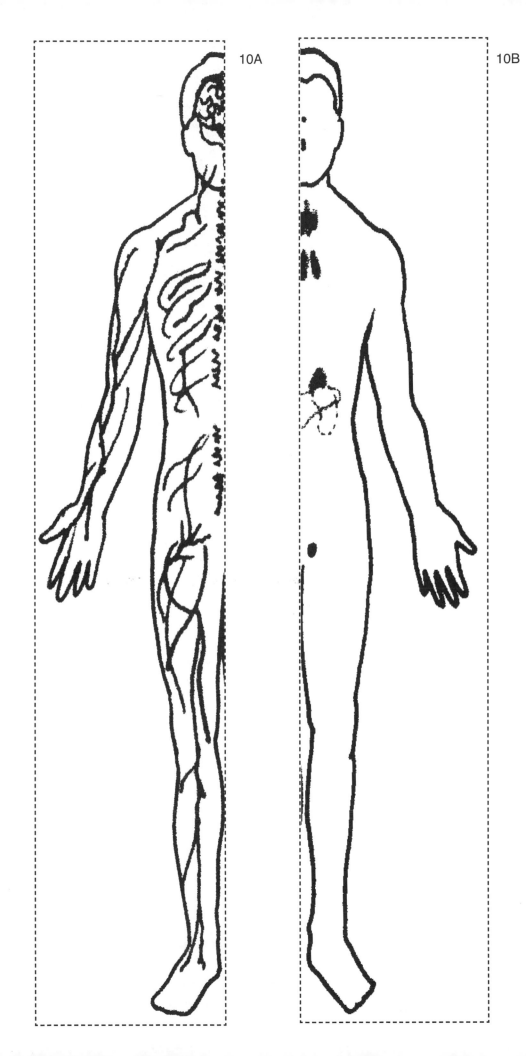

10C

10D

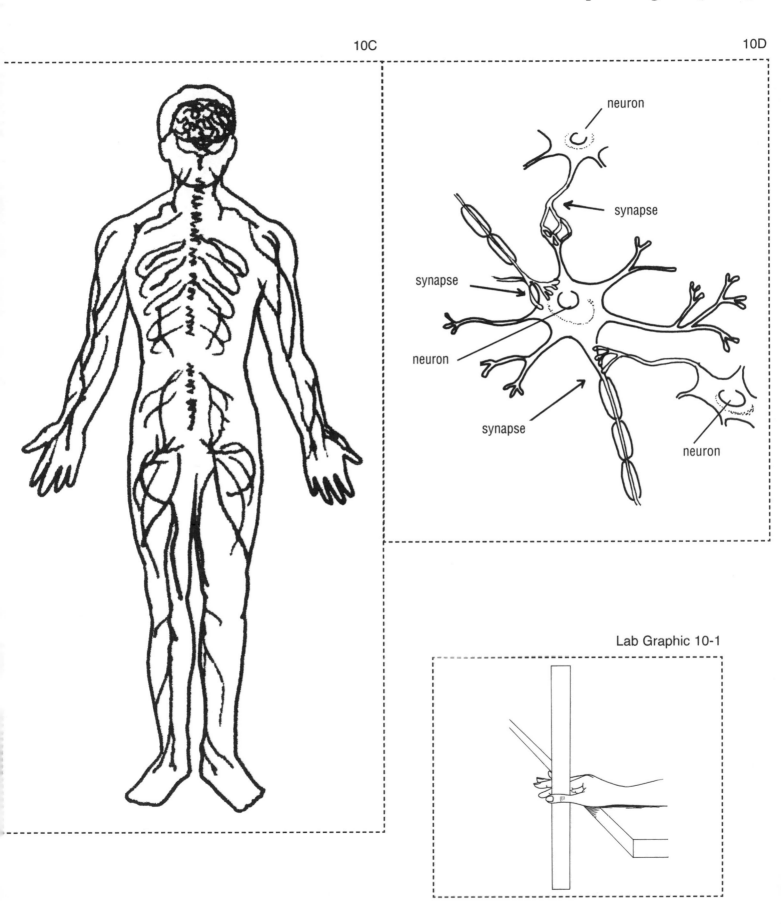

neuron

synapse

synapse

neuron

synapse

neuron

Lab Graphic 10-1

10E

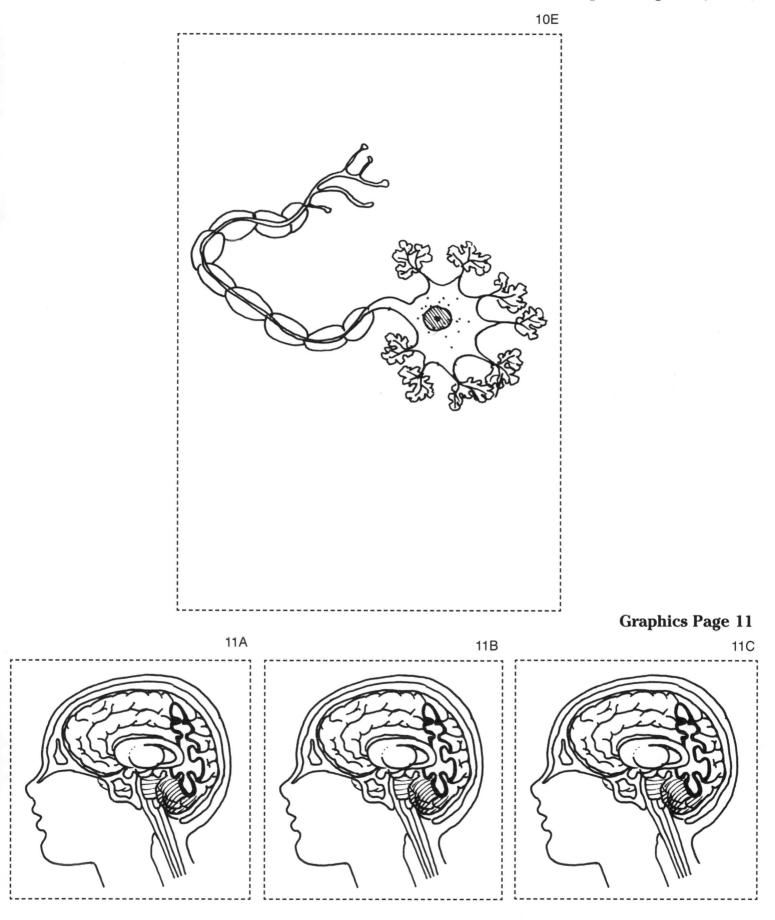

11A

11B

11C

11D

11E

11F

11G

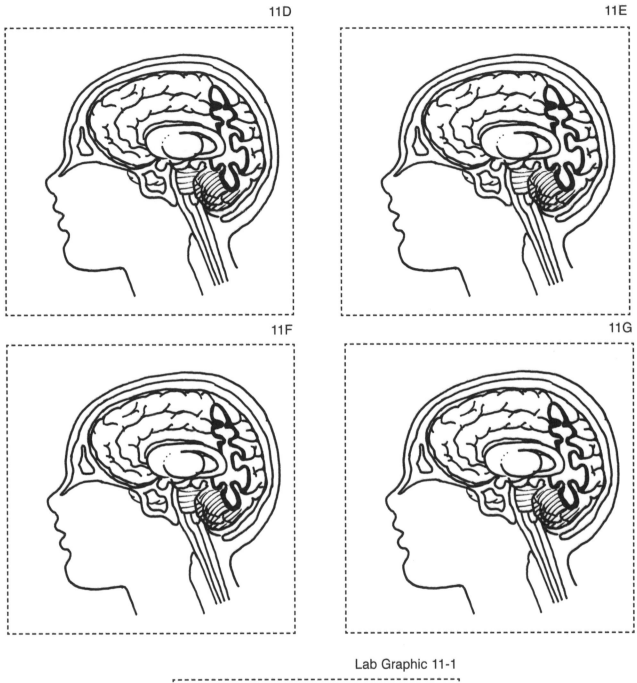

Lab Graphic 11-1

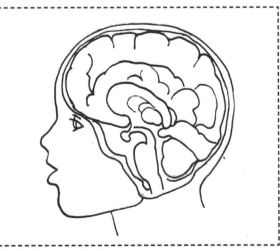

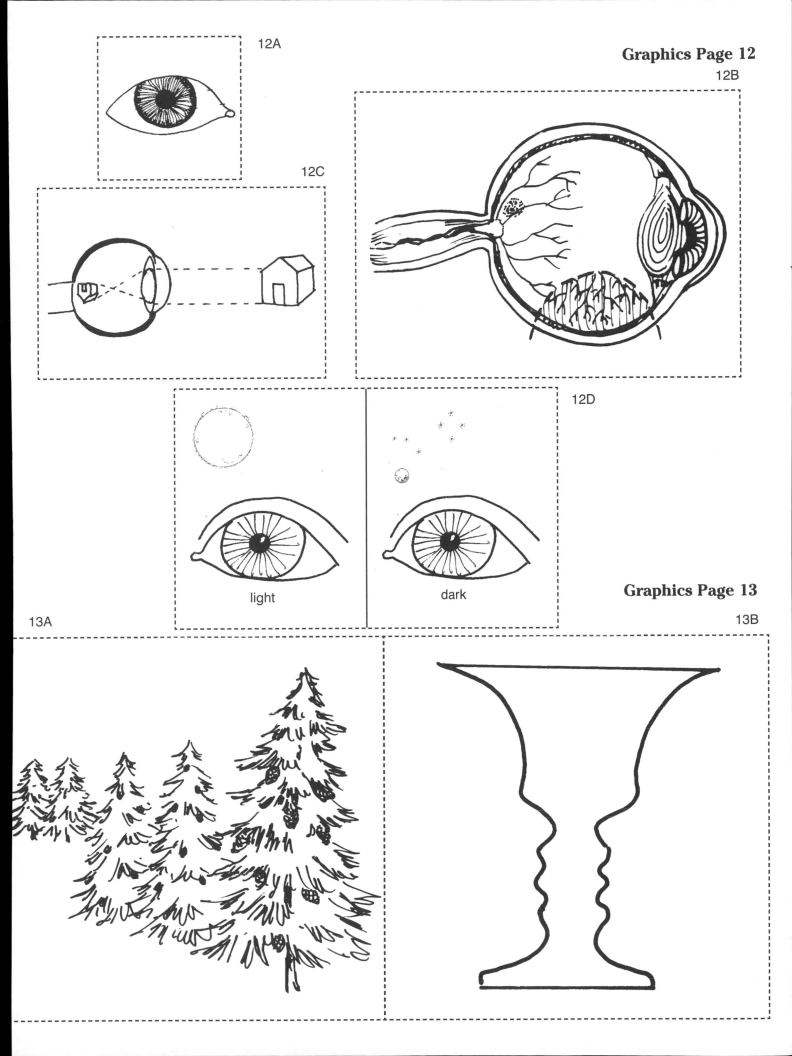

12A

12C

light

dark

12D

13A

13B

13C

13D

13E

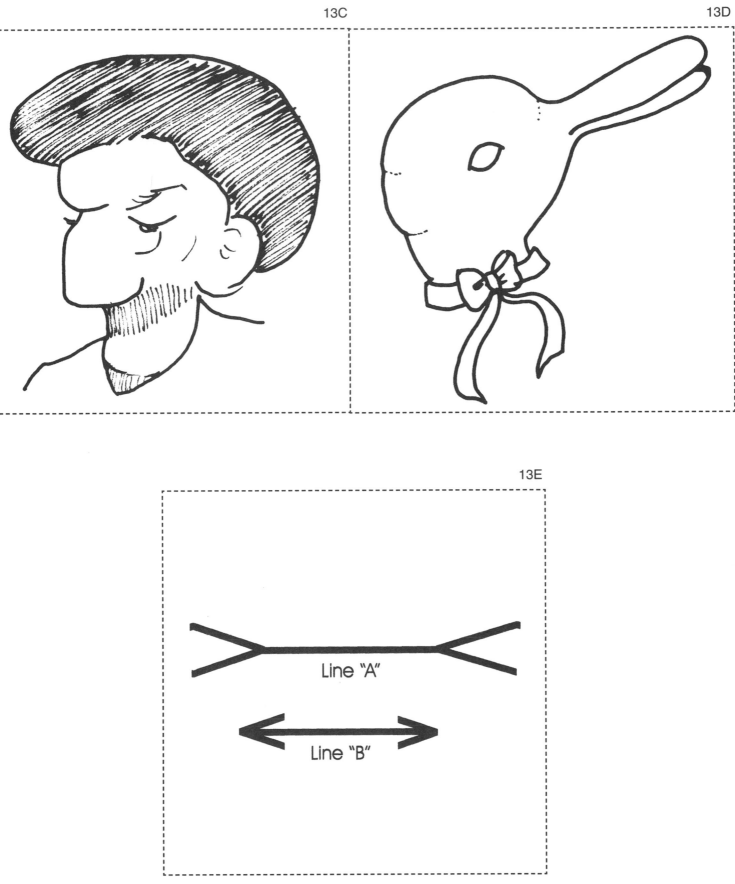

Line "A"

Line "B"

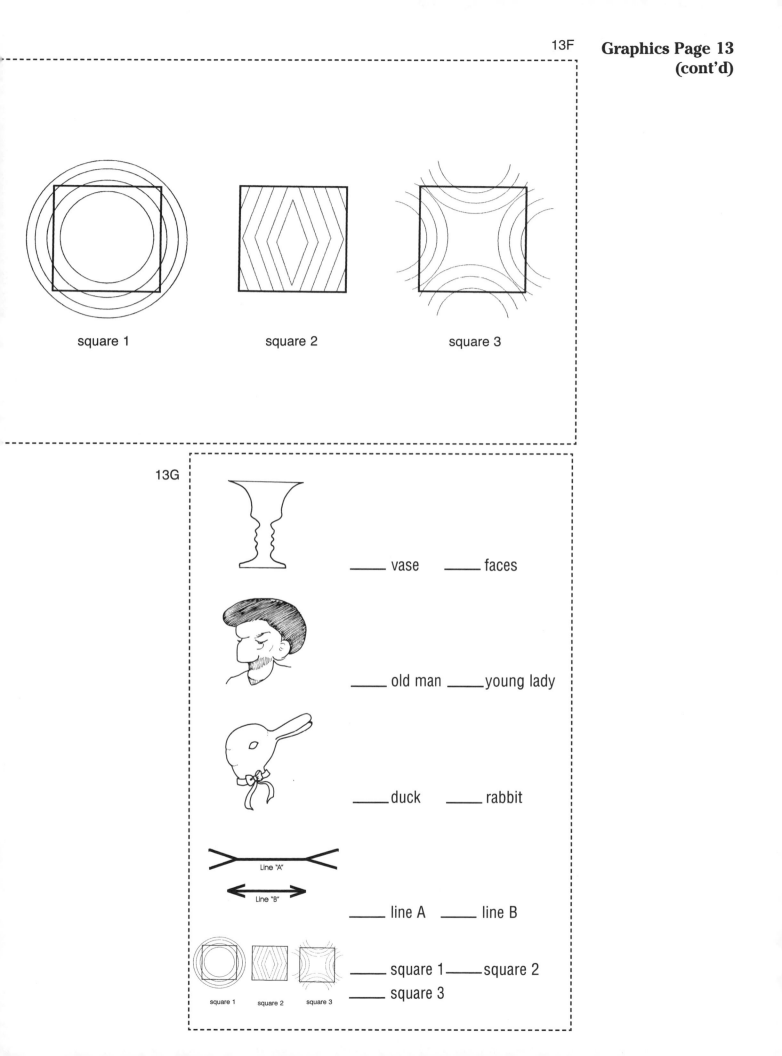

square 1   square 2   square 3

13G

_____ vase   _____ faces

_____ old man _____ young lady

_____ duck   _____ rabbit

Line "A"

Line "B"

_____ line A   _____ line B

_____ square 1 _____ square 2

_____ square 3

14A

14B

14C

14D

low-pitched

Lab Graphic 14-1

catch

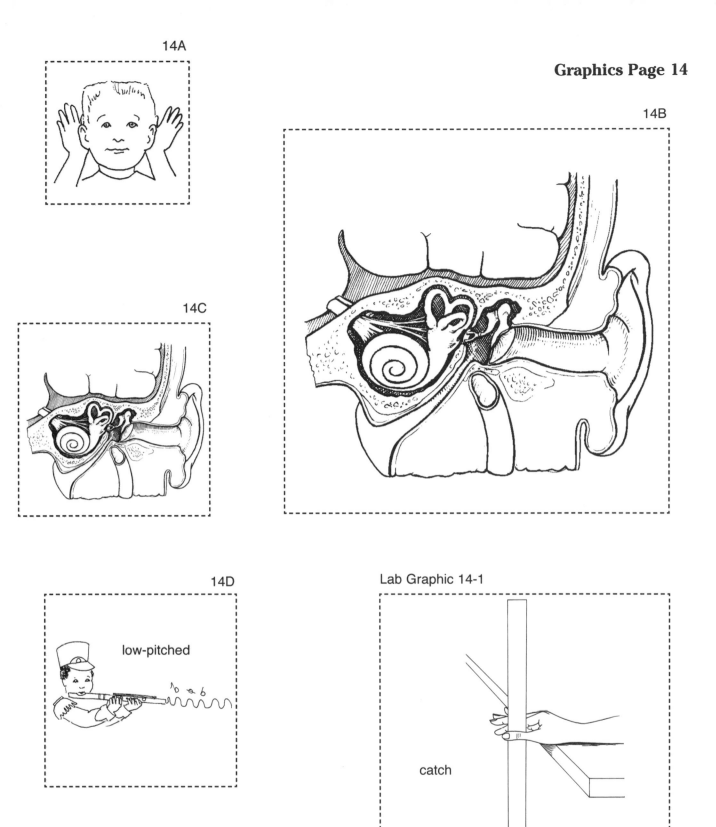

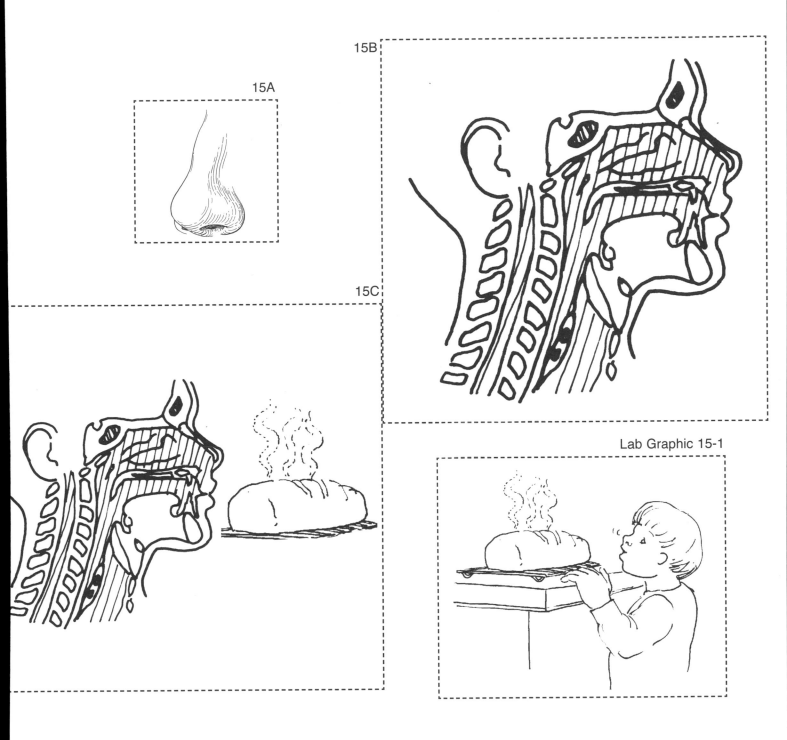

15A

15B

15C

Lab Graphic 15-1

16A

16B

16C

Lab Graphic 16-1

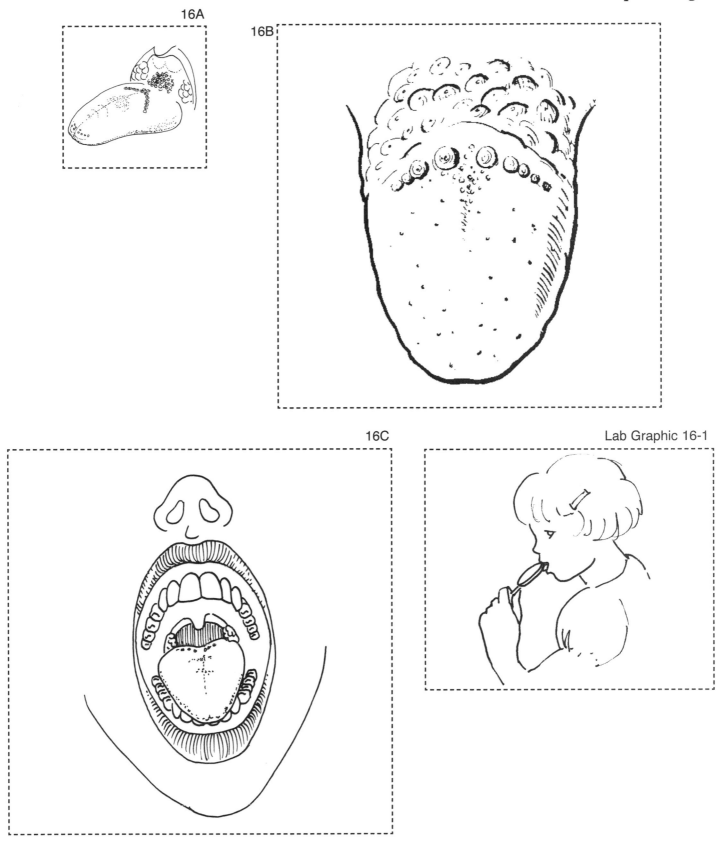

17A

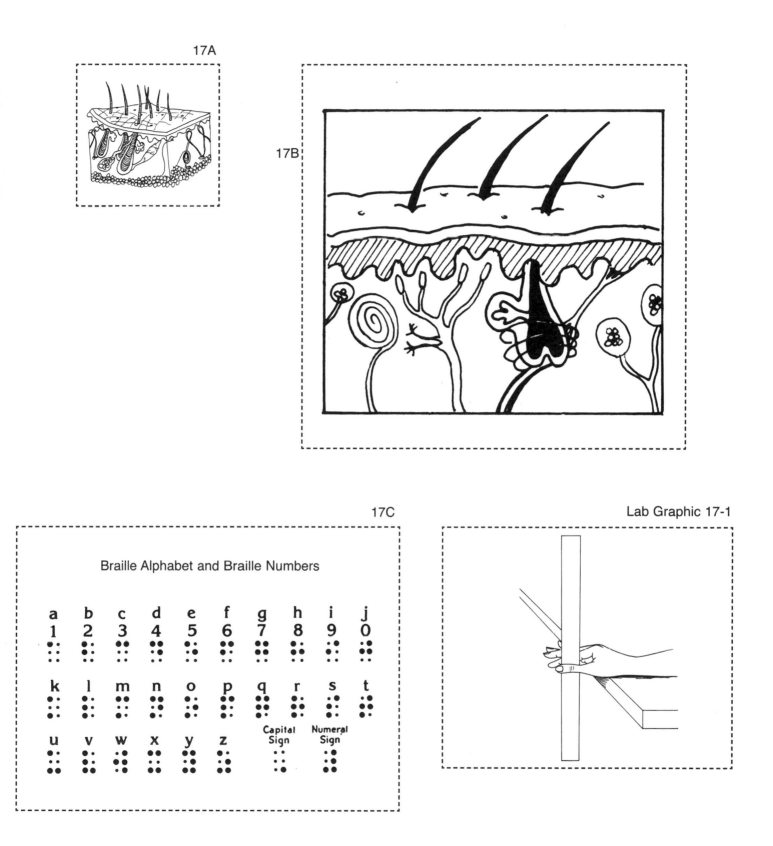

17B

17C

Braille Alphabet and Braille Numbers

Lab Graphic 17-1

18A

18B

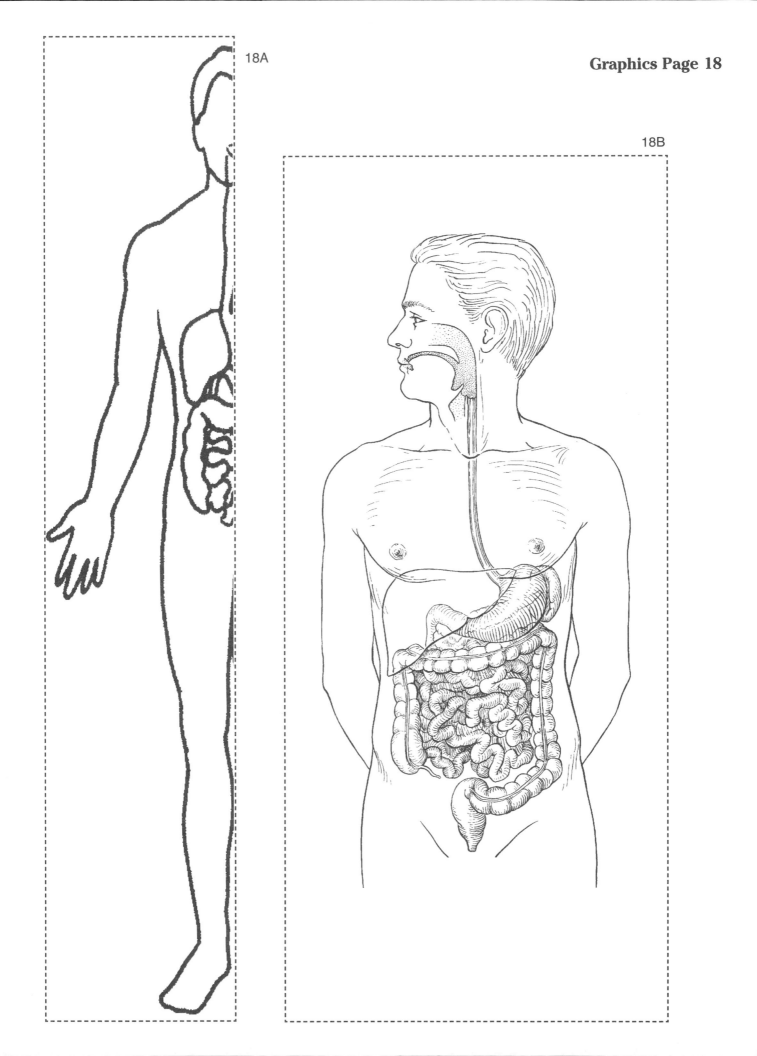

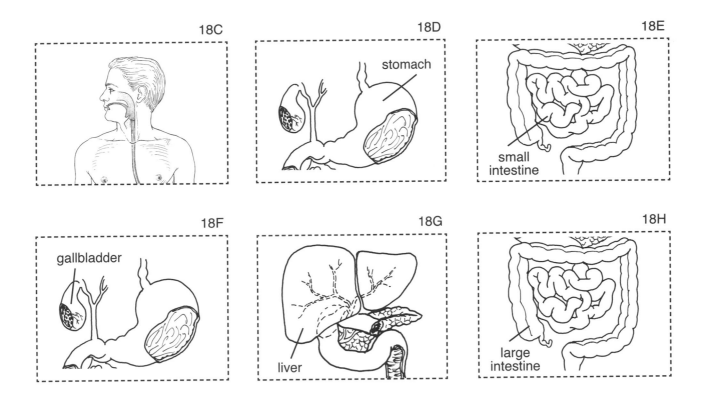

18C

18D
stomach

18E
small
intestine

18F
gallbladder

18G
liver

18H
large
intestine

18I

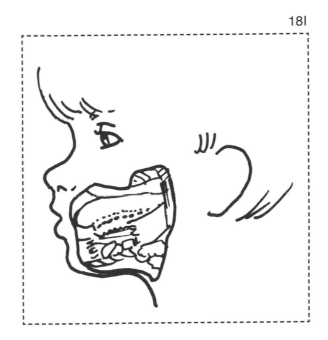

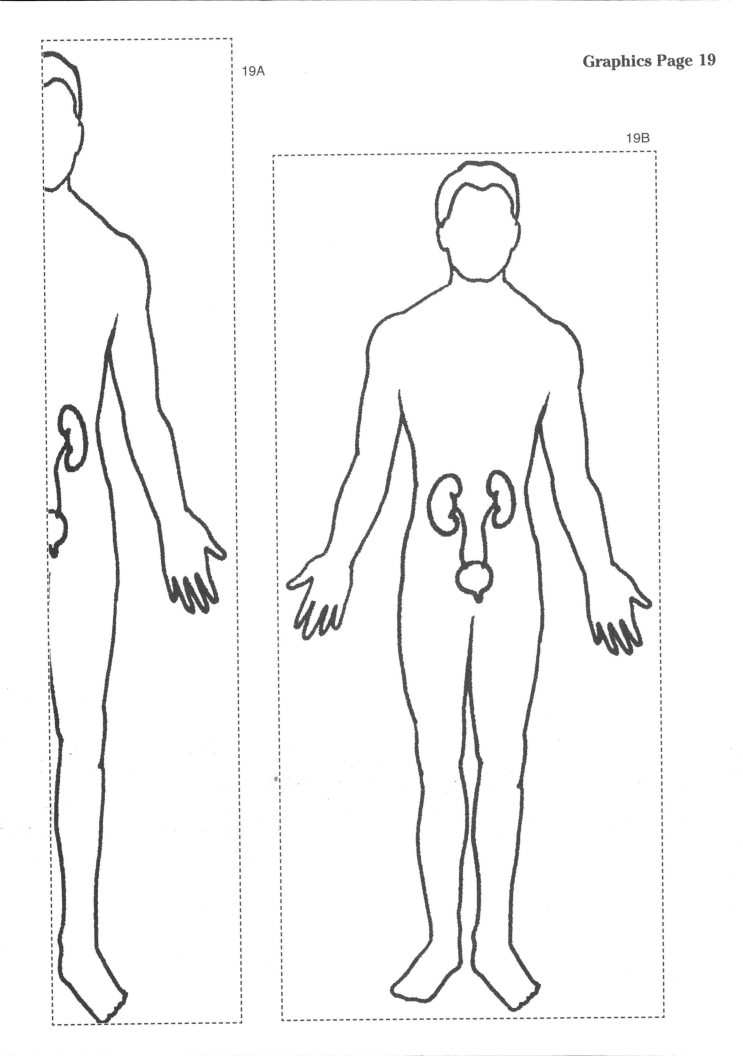

19A

19B

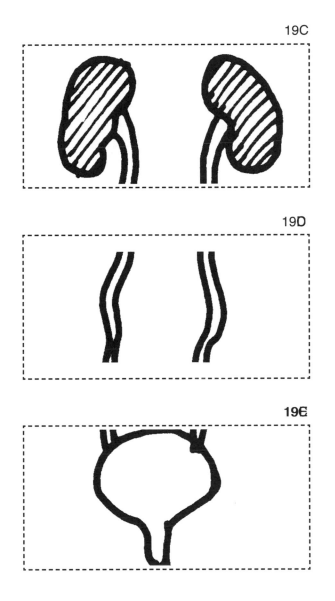

19C

19D

19E

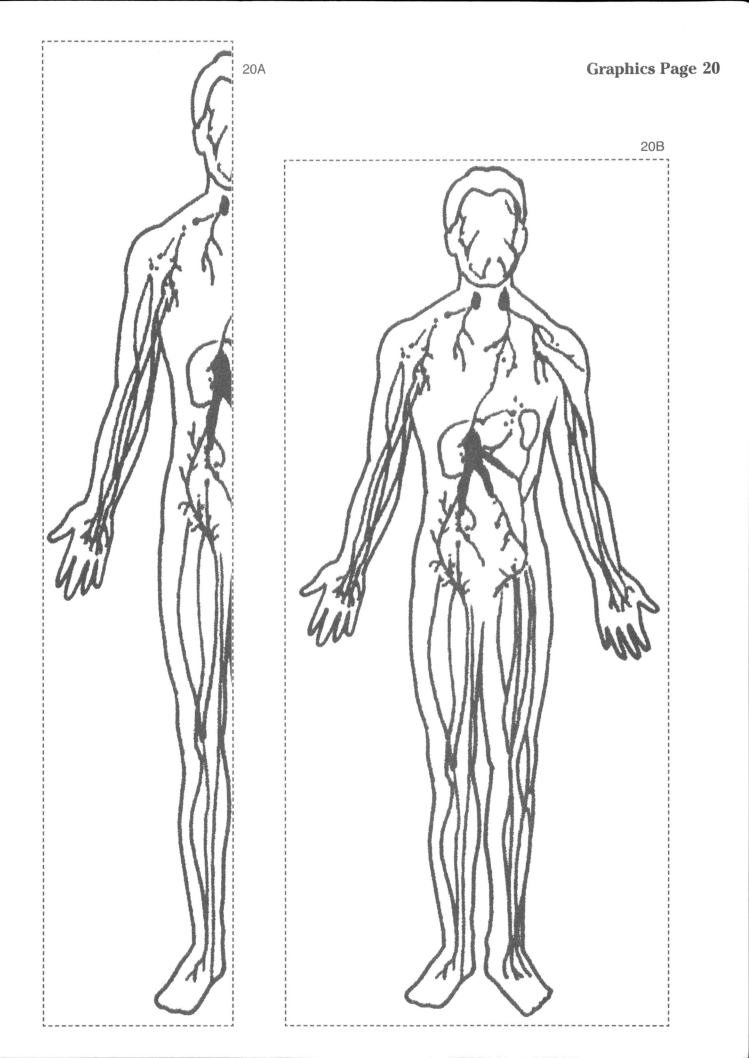

20A

20B

20C

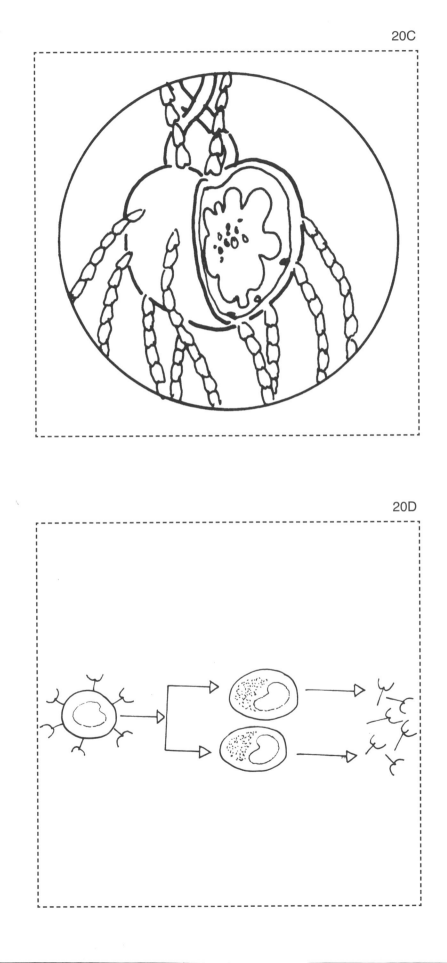

20D

21A

21B

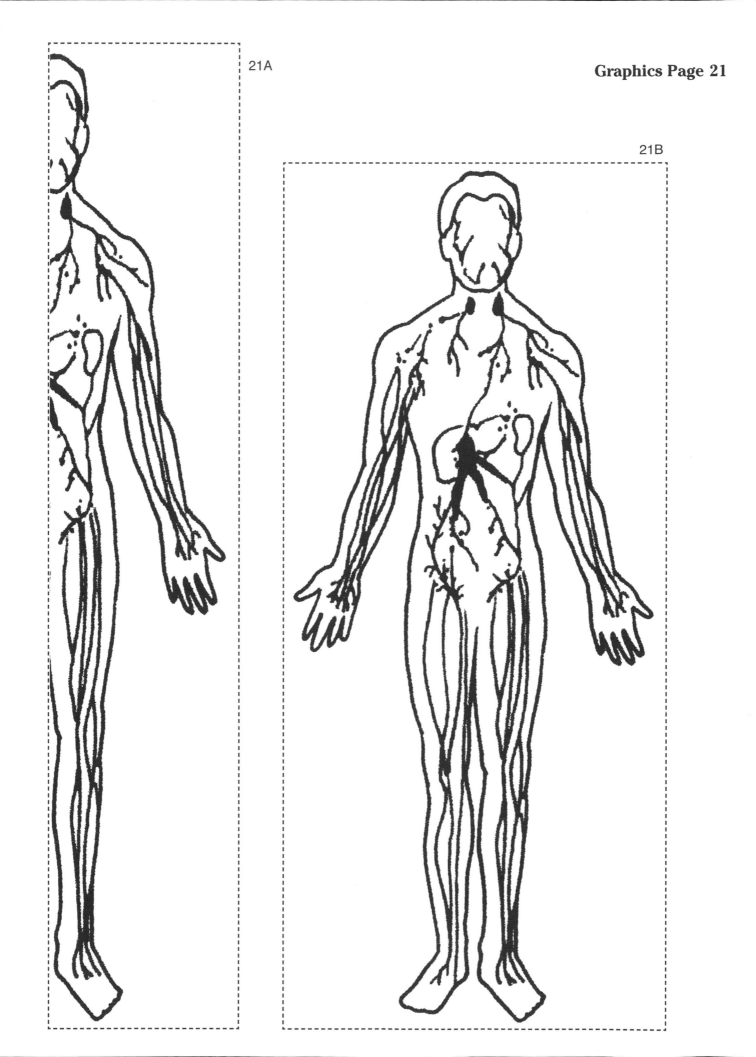

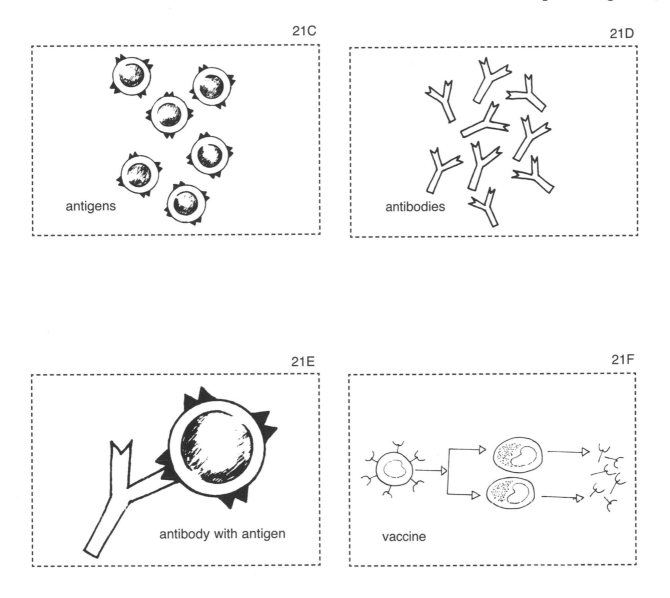

21C antigens

21D antibodies

21E antibody with antigen

21F vaccine

22A

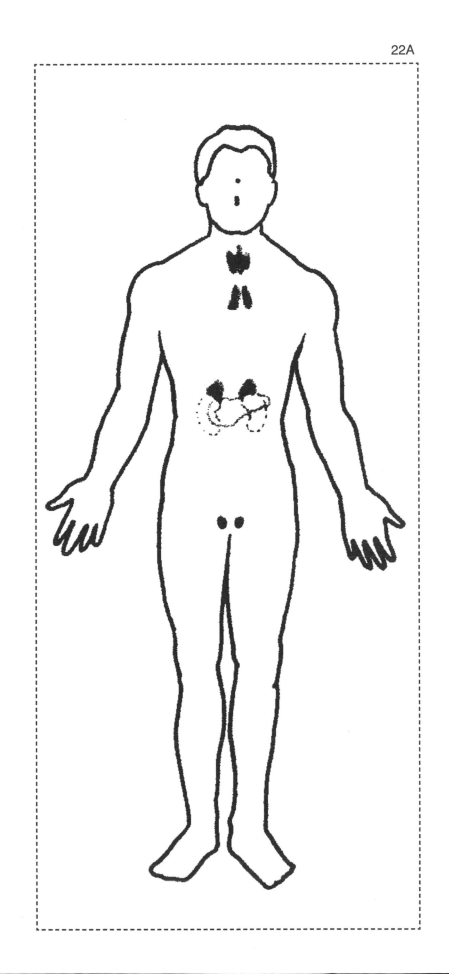

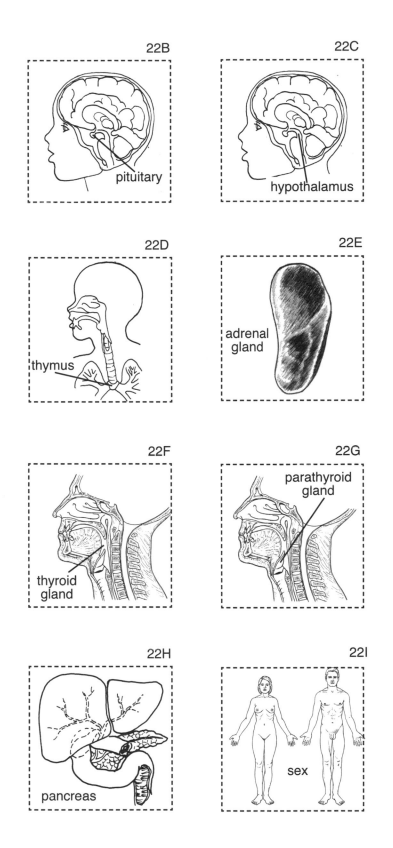

22B

pituitary

22C

hypothalamus

22D

thymus

22E

adrenal gland

22F

thyroid gland

22G

parathyroid gland

22H

pancreas

22I

sex

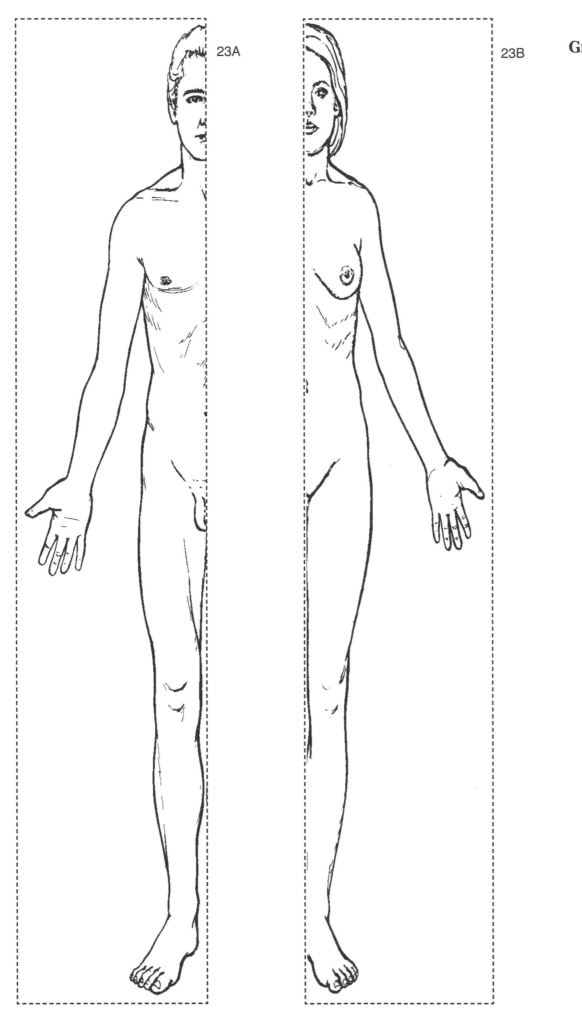

23A

23B

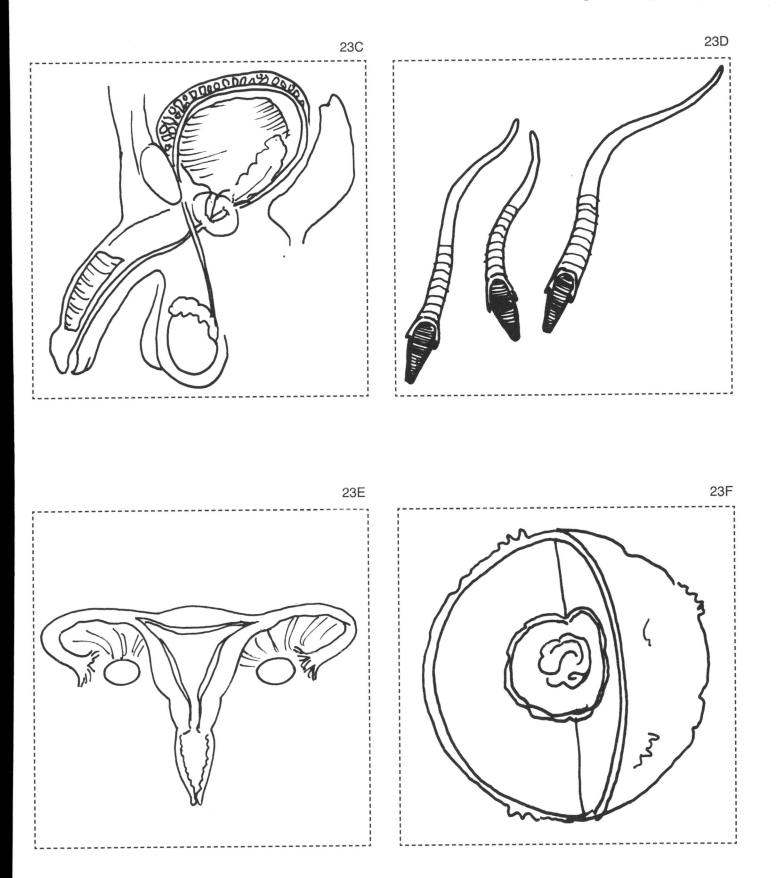

23C

23D

23E

23F

24A

24B

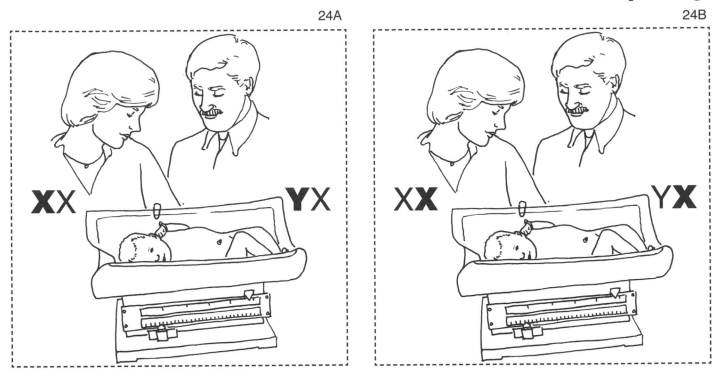

24C

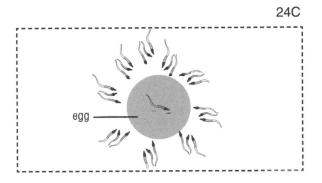

egg

24D

24E

24F

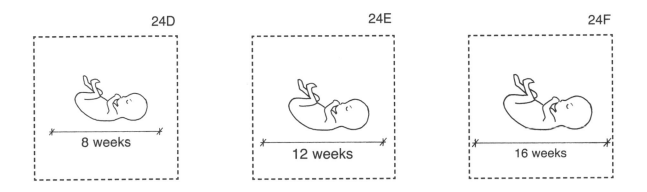

8 weeks

12 weeks

16 weeks

24G

24H

20 weeks

24 weeks

24I

24J

umbilical
cord

amniotic
sac

24K

24L

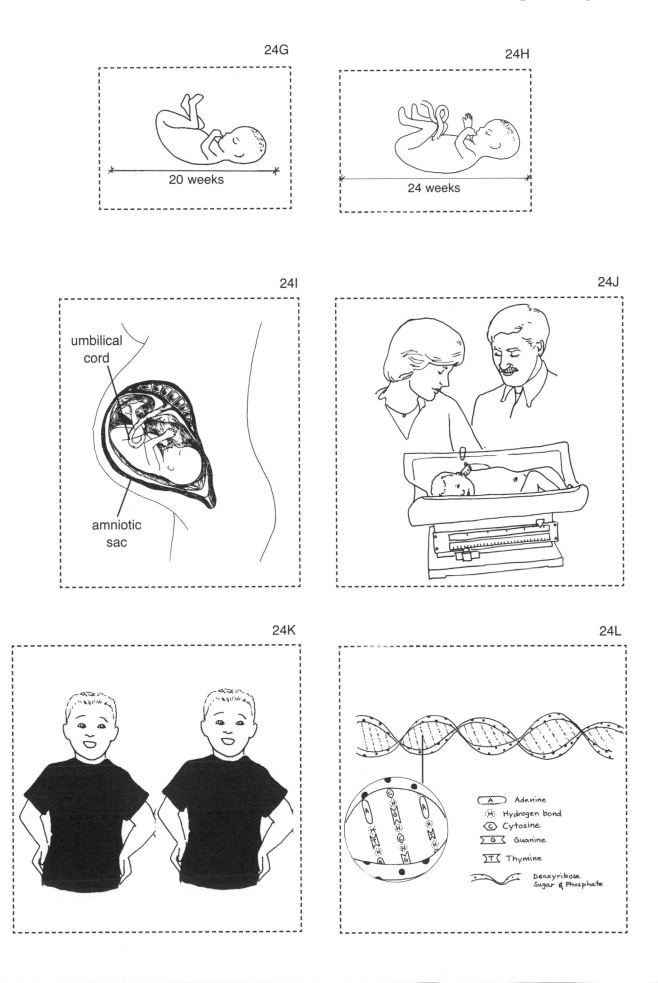